WITHDRAWN

Rehabilitation of

Late-Deafened Adults

Modular Program Manual

Rehabilitation of
Late-Deafened Adults

Modular Program Manual

Jaclyn B. Spitzer, Ph.D.
Chief, Audiology and Speech Pathology Service
VA Medical Center
West Haven, Connecticut
and Associate Clinical Professor
Department of Surgery (Otolaryngology)
Yale University School of Medicine
New Haven, Connecticut

Steven B. Leder, Ph.D.
Associate Professor
Department of Surgery (Otolaryngology)
Yale University School of Medicine
New Haven, Connecticut

Thomas G. Giolas, Ph.D.
Dean, Graduate School
Director, Research Foundation
Professor, Communication Sciences
University of Connecticut
Storrs, Connecticut

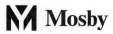 Mosby

St. Louis Baltimore Boston Chicago London Madrid Philadelphia Sydney Toronto

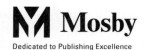

Mosby

Dedicated to Publishing Excellence

Editor: Martha Sasser
Developmental Editor: Barbara S. Menczer
Project Manager: John Rogers
Senior Production Editor: Helen Hudlin
Designer: Julie Taugner
Cover Design: GW Graphics and Publishing
Manufacturing Supervisor: Kathy Grone

Printed in the United States of America
Composition by Clarinda Company
Printing/binding by Maple-Vail Book Mfg. Group

Mosby–Year Book, Inc.
11830 Westline Industrial Drive
St. Louis, Missouri 63146

Library of Congress Cataloging in Publication Data
Spitzer, Jaclyn Barbara.
    Rehabilitation of late-deafened adults : modular program manual /
Jaclyn B. Spitzer, Steven B. Leder, Thomas G. Giolas.   p.   cm.
    Includes bibliographical references and index.
    ISBN 0-8016-7788-2
    1. Postlingual deafness—Patients—Rehabilitation. I. Leder,
Steven B. II. Giolas, Thomas G. III. Title.
    [DNLM: 1. Deafness—rehabilitation. 2. Sensory Aids.   WV 270
S761r 1993]
RF297.S65   1993
617.8′03—dc20
DNLM/DLC   for Library of Congress   93-14225
                                                            CIP

93 94 95 96 97 CL/MY 9 8 7 6 5 4 3 2 1

For E.R., who lived the content of these pages
"For thy sweet love remember'd, such wealth brings
That then I scorn to change my state with kings."

("A Consolation," W. Shakespeare)
Jaclyn B. Spitzer

And to the patients and their families
who participated in this project.

Jaclyn B. Spitzer
Steven B. Leder
Thomas G. Giolas

Acknowledgements

Our program began to evaluate patients for cochlear implant candidacy in 1983. We were, at that time, the sole cochlear implant service in a Veterans Administration medical setting. Funding was provided by the Veteran Administration's Rehabilitation Research and Development Service in Washington, D.C., headed by Dr. Margaret Giannini. We entered into our project development with a sense of discovery and excitement. As we developed our methods, drawing upon the literature, trial and error, and common sense, our cochlear implant team evolved into a cohesive and creative unit.

We were fortunate from the outset to have the support of clinicians with extensive clinical experience with deafness: Frederick Richardson, M.D., Chief of Rehabilitation Medicine at VAMC West Haven, and Clarence T. Sasaki, M.D., Chairman of Otolaryngology at Yale University School of Medicine. Their interest in developing a cochlear implant program with both clinical and research activity led to my (J. Spitzer) coming to Connecticut in 1982. Their administrative support and insight were of assistance throughout the early phases of the program and continue today. Administrative guidance was also provided by the Director of Audiology and Speech Pathology Service at the Department of Veterans Affairs' Central Office in Washington, D.C., Henry Speuhler, Ph.D. Currently, his successor, Allen Boysen, Ph.D., is taking an active interest in the establishment of a clinical cochlear implant program policy for the VA system, thus allowing us fruitful discussion of the practical issues involved in providing services to deaf and hearing-impaired veterans and other late-deafened adults.

The team of audiologists and speech-language pathologists involved in our project included Carole Flevaris-Phillips, Ph.D.; Myles A. Kessler, M.A.; Steven B. Leder, Ph.D.; Nancy McMahon, M.A.; Paul Milner, Ph.D.; Martha Rubin, Ed.D.; Marilyn Russell, Ph.D.; and Mary Murray, Program Coordinator. Thomas G. Giolas, Ph.D., was a consultant from the program's inception. These people contributed their expertise, creativity, and insights derived from diverse backgrounds to make the project an enjoyable exploration of our capabilities in evaluational and rehabilitative methods.

The otolaryngologists participating in the team were Linda Gardiner, M.D., and J. Cameron Kirchner, M.D., both enthusiastic supporters of the surgical and follow-up phases of patient care. Our investigational and clinical activity continues today with John F. Kveton, M.D.

The neuropsychologist evaluating our patients was Richard Delaney, Ph.D. The caseload provided him with challenging individuals both from a technical and interpretive perspective. Our statistical support was provided, often late into the evening, by Emanuel Lerner, M.A.

For each of the authors, development of this book would have been impossible had it not been for the understanding and encouragement of our families. They not only put up with our long hours, but they fed us too.

J.B.S.

Contents

Rehabilitation of
Late-Deafened Adults

Modular Program Manual

CHAPTER 1

Rehabilitation of the Late-Deafened Adult: An Overview and Philosophy

TECHNOLOGY has burst on the health scene with numerous innovations for the physically and sensorially impaired—amputees are now able to ski, wheelchair users to race, and speech and language impaired to communicate using computers. The quality of life for many persons has been altered in ways not envisioned 10 years ago. These developments have captured the public's imagination and raised awareness.

Technologic advances have made a dramatic impact on the treatment of individuals with sensory impairment. Scanners now read books for the visually impaired and transcribe text both into and from Braille with fluidity. Similar advances have affected the quality of life for the hearing impaired. Improvements in quality and size of components have taken hearing aids and assistive listening devices light years from their crude inception. In an almost science fiction–like manner, the field of deafness has been transformed by the introduction of implantable devices and sophisticated vibrotactile aids.

There is a gap, however, between the promise that such technology offers to the profoundly hearing-impaired person and the actuality of the perceived benefit and service delivery. The shortfall is clearly demonstrated in the need for legislation to mandate equal access to the communicative tools of our society. The enactment of the Americans with Disabilities Act of 1991 reflects recognition of the present lack of access for the disabled and establishes requirements for achieving technologic equality of access in both the public and private sectors. Extending the aims of the Rehabilitation Act of 1973, the Americans with Disabilities Act prohibits discrimination based on disability in employment, public accommodations, transportation, and telecommunications (Bebout, 1991). It is anticipated that the act will have an impact on auditory accessibility and will lead to increased use of assistive devices for the hearing impaired in public places such as classrooms, conference rooms, and theaters. However, since we have not yet seen the fruits (nor the enabling regulations) of this law, we cannot discuss whether it will, as hoped, bridge the gap for the hearing impaired.

Acknowledging that there are societal gaps in the accessibility and application of new technology for the hearing impaired, we must also recognize that there are gaps in the provision of rehabilitative services for this group. In some cases, the need for intervention has been minimized (some findings have shown that persons with adult-onset hearing loss have normal voice or articulatory production [Espir and Rose, 1976; Goehl and Kaufman, 1984; Ling, 1976]) without looking at such critical factors as length of deafness or history of (or current) hearing aid usage. When the latter factors are included in analyses, it is clear that some individuals with profound hearing loss do indeed have therapeutic needs (Leder and Spitzer, 1990). Therefore global statements about the rehabilitative need of persons with late-onset deafness are probably not appropriate, and individual assessment is necessary to devise therapy plans.

We know that the devices used—whether auditory, tactile, or implanted electrical—provide awareness and signal detection, yet the recognition of sounds and speech may not easily be obtained. Such devices offer the promise of hearing restoration or new stimulation which, without guidance and training, may elude the user. Into this breach the audiologist, speech-language pathologist, or teacher of the hearing impaired must go to serve as a guide to help the user reach his/her full potential benefit.

THERAPEUTIC MILIEU

The atmosphere within which a rehabilitative program develops often reflects its underlying philosophy. The isolated involvement of one or two professionals without consultation and cross-validation of their assessment and practices is not the optimal situation for attaining therapeutic goals or professional function. Often a clinician faces a late-deafened adult, as a first such case for aural rehabilitation, with a sense of dread and insecurity, despite the necessary academic preparation. Acknowledging that special qualifications and competencies for aural rehabilitation have been defined (Committee on Aural Rehabilitation, ASHA, 1984), there is still a further subset of training and experience not common to all clinicians that is necessary for working with the target group. Often lack of experience in training procedures for a specific assistive device (such as a multichannel vibrotactile aid) poses difficulty.

In an idealized setting, a team should be involved in the evaluational and rehablitative care of a hearing-impaired adult. However, when it is not possible to confer in person with other specialists in the field of aural rehabilitation, it is often beneficial to develop "long distance" consultations with such peers and/or experts;

such sharing of case information can permit confirmation of conclusions or can provide new insights into solving aural rehabilitative challenges.

When undertaken, development of a team approach provides the opportunity to share diversified viewpoints regarding a given patient's needs and generates well-rounded therapeutic goals. A team may consist of many individuals whose involvement differs at different stages of assessment or treatment. The specialties of audiology, speech-language pathology, psychology, otolaryngology, rehabilitation medicine, optometry, and social work may all be involved to a different extent. Subspecialties of aural rehabilitation and psychoacoustics may be needed (Leder et al., 1987). Availability of consultation and referral to such resources as vocational counselors for the deaf, vocational training facilities, and interpreter services can greatly enhance program outcomes.

In some settings, a team is gathered with the narrow purpose of developing a cochlear implant program. However, frequently, the team recognizes that patients and families inquiring about a particular form of treatment, such as implantation, in fact would be better served if broader rehabilitative needs were addressed.

DEVELOPMENT OF A METHOD

This manual presents the organized results of our aural rehabilitation team who developed training procedures and rehabilitative counseling that were needed by many of our prospective candidates, implant users, and noncandidates. Although we began as an implant team, we quickly found that our patients' needs demanded a broader clinical approach. In fact, despite heavy pre-admission screening, we found that fewer than 20% of the patients evaluated were really appropriate for implantation; yet 100% had auditory, communicative, and psychologic problems that needed to be addressed.

This book is the result of an evolution in our practice and presents training procedures developed by our rehabilitation team, expanding on our objectives in working with severely and profoundly hearing-impaired adults. We describe procedures we found to be useful with persons who were not implant candidates but for whom the isolation and communicative impact of severe or profound late-onset deafness had, nonetheless, imposed considerable obstacles.

TERMINOLOGY AND TARGET PATIENTS

Several terms in this text will be used interchangeably. To describe our patients' impairment, we have chosen the term *late-onset deafness* or *hearing loss*, which has gained broad usage. We use the latter term as synonymous with *adventitious, post-lingual, post-linguistic onset,* or *adult-onset hearing loss* although we recognize that there may be nuances of meaning among these appellations. For example, a person may be adventitiously or post-linguistically impaired during childhood as well as later in life.

The persons who are intended to participate in this therapy program are *profoundly* hearing-impaired adults (audiometric thresholds of 90 dB Hearing Level [HL]) whose loss occurred after language acquisition. They may be (1) cochlear implant candidates or persons previously implanted, (2) hearing aid users who are not presently candidates for implantation but who are attempting to maximize their aided performance and social adjustment, or (3) users of vibrotactile devices rather than auditory stimulation. This program has application as well to (4) persons with *severe* hearing impairment (audiometric thresholds of 75 to 85 dB HL) whose present skill level and/or adjustment are deemed suboptimal. Persons whose severe hearing loss appears to be progressive may benefit from training while residual hearing permits acquisition of skills and integration of stimulation.

As the field of cochlear implantation continues to advance, the criteria for selection of candidates may also evolve to include persons with less-than-profound hearing loss. The definition of lack of benefit from a hearing aid may also change in the future. Another alteration in candidate selection may occur as persons undergoing removal of acoustic tumors are implanted with electrode(s) into the cochlear nucleus (Eisenberg et al., 1987) and are provided with increasingly sophisticated, multichannel stimulation (Luetje et al., 1992).

The current criteria for cochlear implantation are listed in the box below. These criteria are comparable to those described elsewhere (Clark et al., 1977; House and Berliner, 1982; Mecklenberg and Brimacombe, 1985; Simmons, 1985). The latter criteria were applied in accepting referrals to our program, which led to the development of our database and quartile ranges.

CRITERIA FOR COCHLEAR IMPLANTATION*

- Profound bilateral sensorineural hearing loss
- No response to brainstem auditory-evoked potentials
- Severe impairment of speech discrimination and recognition performance
- Adult between 18 and 70 years of age
- Ability to tolerate surgery
- Normal temporal bone findings
- Normal psychologic examination
- Understanding of possible benefits and limitations of implantation

---

*See text for further discussion of current criteria for implantation and rehabilitation.
Modified from Spitzer JB: *VA Practitioner* 3:50-52, 1986.

TABLE 1-1   Patient pool characteristics (N = 34)

Characteristic	$\overline{X}$	SD
Age	53	13.64
Age at time of hearing loss	26.47	13.42
Hearing loss (# of years)	15.91	13.41
Education (# of years)	12.21	2.96 (range = 8-18)

Tables 1-1 and 1-2 summarize the historical background of the first 34 patients seen in our program. The predominant number of males reflects the VA population. Most striking is the wide variety of etiologic factors that affected their hearing. In addition, an interesting observation that we initially thought might influence our rehabilitative planning (see Chapter 2) was the number of patients whose background included a serious head injury (e.g., motor vehicle accident) or other central nervous system insult (e.g., meningitis). Table 1-3 summarizes the patients' unaided and (hearing) aided audiometric profile.

We learned early in our program not to assume that patients who come to a deafness rehabilitation center are adequately fitted with proper assistive devices. The following example—actually a case of good hearing aid fitting—illustrates this point.

CASE STUDY 1.1

From a small town in upstate Georgia, D.D. lost his hearing to ototoxic drugs used to treat tuberculosis at the end of World War II. He had received consistent care from Audiology Services in the VA since his discharge. Numerous hearing aid arrangements had been tried, with minimal success in his overall communicative performance. He arrived at our door wearing two powerful body aids, which he had obtained from his local VA medical center. During the previous 10 years, he had received lipreading training several times.

He attempted unsuccessfully to wear his binaural arrangement but often complained of dizziness when wearing both body aids. His communicative performance was poor with the latter set-up. He and his wife were very frustrated with their day-to-day communication.

After evaluation, we found he had sufficient residual hearing (Table 1-4) to permit use of binaural behind-the-ear hearing aids. Although he persistently struggled to maintain sufficiently tight earmolds to eliminate feedback, the advantage of true binaural ear-level input resulted in better face-to-face communication. He required additional training to improve his visual attentiveness and lipreading strategies. Several auditory and other communicative measures (Table 1-4) showed improvement after an intensive course of therapy.

The severely and profoundly hearing-impaired adult has, in our experience often been told, sometimes in the distant past, that his/her hearing loss was too

TABLE 1-2   Historical background of patients referred for rehabilitation
(N = 34)

Subject	Age at evaluation (yrs)	Gender	Age of onset (yrs)	Duration of profound loss (yrs)	Probable etiology
1	60	M	19	41	Meningitis
2	49	M	34	15	Unknown
3	54	M	33	23	Noise +
4	61	M	12	7	Otosclerosis
5	36	F	29	32	Familial (?)
6	65	M	30	5	Otosclerosis
7	68	M	30	18	Noise +
8	64	M	31	33	Systemic infection
9	20	M	5	15	Unknown
10	42	M	38	3	Meningitis
11	63	M	32	30	Otosclerosis
12	59	M	37	22	Sudden hearing loss (ototoxicity?)
13	61	M	19	1	Syphilis
14	58	M	18	40	Noise +
15	44	M	38	9	Unknown
16	66	M	20	36	Ototoxicity
17	66	M	24	4	Noise +
18	57	M	18	36	Noise +
20	54	M	19	19	Noise +
20	45	M	37	8	Struck by lightning
21	69	M	29	3	Familial
22	65	F	28	45	Ototoxicity and familial
23	66	M	64	2	Meningitis
24	20	M	5	2	Unknown
25	59	M	18	21	Meningitis
26	49	M	19	4	Fungal infections
27	47	M	8	31	Otitis media
28	26	F	21	5	Meningitis
29	60	M	34	15	Unknown
30	68	M	56	12	Ototoxicity
31	64	M	24	6	MVA
32	56	M	47	7	Skull fracture; meningitis
33	33	M	25	8	MVA
34	49	M	24	25	Ototoxicity (kidney failure)

Noise + = progressive loss with other possible influences that cannot be determined adequately.
MVA = motor vehicle accident.

TABLE 1-3   Unaided and aided audiometric profile of patients referred (N = 34)

Subject	3 frequency pure-tone average (PTA)—better ear unaided (dB HL)	3 frequency pure-tone average (PTA)—better ear aided (dB HL)
1	125+	110+
2	125+	110+
3	125+	110+
4	125+	110+
5	125+	110+
6	113v	60
7	90	52
8	112v	53
9	117	85
10	125+	104v
11	105	60
12	125+	110+
13	95	57
14	112	56
15	98v	55
16	107v	51
17	114v	110+
18	125+	92v
19	125+	110+
20	98v	55
21	97v	49
22	125+	109v
23	125+	110+
24	125+	80
25	125+	92v
26	125+	110+
27	125+	110+
28	125+	90
29	125+	110+
30	110	59
31	125+	110+
32	125+	79
33	125+	78
34	125+	71

+ indicates that response exceeded audiometric limits under headphones (unaided) or in sound field (aided).

v indicates that patient-reported response was at least partially (or totally) vibrotactile in nature.

TABLE 1-4 Summary of D.D.'s performance after hearing aid fitting and intensive rehabilitation

Test	Initial score	Post-treatment score*
Pure-Tone Average (PTA)† (3 frequency) with headphones		
Right	108	103
Left	106	108
Speech Detection Threshold (SDT)†		
Right	92	DNT‡
Left	86	DNT
PTA (3 frequency)†		
Aided	49 (body aid, right)	38 (binaural behind-the-ears)
SDT		
Aided†	45 (″)	25 (″)
Monosyllable-Trochee-Spondee (MTS)		
Words correct	12	12‡
Stress correct	19	20‡
West Haven Speechreading Battery (% correct)		
NAL-West Haven	12	46
Iowa-Keaster	14	70
CID Sentences (5 lists)	0-6	12-30
Gold Rush	0	0‡

DNT–did not test.
*Follow-up 10 months after initial evaluation.
†In dB hearing level (HL) re: American National Standards Institute (ANSI) 1970.
‡No change from initial test score to retest score.

great to allow use of a hearing aid and that he/she was beyond help. Given this information, at some point in time efforts to obtain help may cease or diminish, and, worse yet, attempts to seek information may stop entirely. It is difficult to obtain information, even if some spark of hope survives, because such adults do not have the necessary resources such as the specialized devices for the deaf (tele-caption decoders, telecommunication devices [TDDs], FM auditory trainers, and other assistive devices), which have been introduced since they lost contact with more recent developments.

Therefore it is not surprising that, when a center announces it is beginning a new program to help the deaf, a flood of inquiries from hearing-impaired persons, family, or friends result and that many of these people have poor or very outdated information about treatment of the hearing impaired. This experience has been

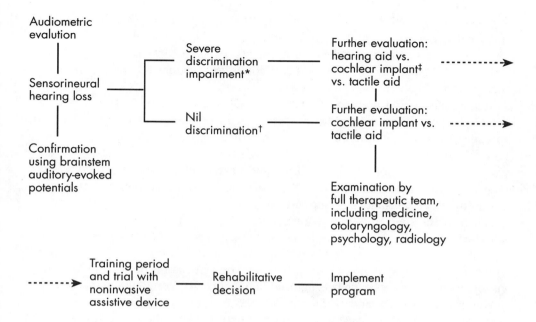

*Changing criteria for definition of "severe" speech discrimination impairment. Presently, investigational studies only are permitted to implant persons with discrimination ≤ 20%.

†Traditional requirement for cochlear implanation has been speech discrimination ≤ 2% (NU=6 words).

‡In this scenario, use of a cochlear implant would imply investigational use in view of some residual speech discrimination.

Fig. 1-1. Flow of assessment toward rehabilitative decision.

shared by many centers when they begin to advertise that they are offering cochlear implant services. Many of the persons inquiring, while not necessarily appropriate cochlear implant candidates, are indeed persons for whom a rehabilitation program for the late-deafened adult can render important services.

REHABILITATIVE ASSESSMENT

Assessment of the rehabilitative needs of a severely or profoundly hearing-impaired adult proceeds in a stepwise manner, as illustrated in Fig. 1-1. After thorough audiometric evaluation and confirmation of the level of hearing impairment by an objective method (e.g., Brainstem Auditory-Evoked Potentials), a protocol is initiated to delineate the extent of benefit obtained from the presently used assistive device as well as from some possibly advantageous device that may be technologically superior or employ a different modality. Such evaluation includes psychoacoustic and communicative measurements, which lead to the development of a picture of the patient's abilities and limitations. Suggestions for specific measurements are highlighted in each chapter of this text.

Examination by a number of other specialists is warranted (Spitzer, 1986; Leder et al., 1987). Tyler, Tye-Murray, and Gantz (1991) similarly emphasize that specialists in assessment of communicative function (for hearing and vision limitations, verbal and manual language ability), psychology, vocational needs, and physical skills (for mobility, upper limb, and dexterity limitations) should participate in the evaluation. The place of the audiologic examination in the larger evaluation by other specialities is shown in Fig. 1-2.

Each of the specialists may contribute significantly to the overall care of the late-deafened adult as well as to the rehabilitative decision. For example, we came to understand the importance of including an optometrist on our team because a number of our patients had visual problems. The association of hearing loss with visual disorders has been well-recognized in patients with congenital or early-onset deafness (Konigsmark and Gorlin, 1976) and in the geriatric population (Kline and Schieber, 1985). However, in a group of persons with late-onset deafness, the association had not been formally documented. In our sample, we (Spitzer and Perlin, unpublished) found a substantial need for optometric evaluation and intervention as a necessary precursor to proceeding with a full rehabilitative assessment and plan. Specifically, 22 (64.7%) of our sample patients required a new prescription for eyeglasses and two (5.8%) needed a new prescription for reading tasks. Only three (8.8%) did not need eyeglasses at all, while five (14.7%) came to the program appropriately fit visually. Two (5.8%) were uncooperative or could not follow instructions sufficiently to complete the examination. The optometrist also discussed with our patients the possibility of assistance in long-distance lip-reading through use of a monocular telescope, a suggestion pursued by eight (23.5%) in the group. In view of our program's interest in improving communication through visual input, in conjunction with an assistive device, and the heavy reliance on written and/or videotaped counselling materials, a required change of prescription for a total of 24 (70.5%) of our group highlighted the need for involvement of an optometric specialist.

Upon completed evaluation by the other subspecialities, an experimental course of (audiologic) training and an ensuing trial period with an assistive listening device (ALD) of a noninvasive nature (hearing aid with ALD or vibrotactile aid) should be carried out. Progress with this device should be assessed further.

At this point, it may be determined that progress with an auditory input is poor or unlikely. If no progress is measured in an adult after such training, alternative stimulation methods (vibrotactile or electrical) may be considered. The therapeu-

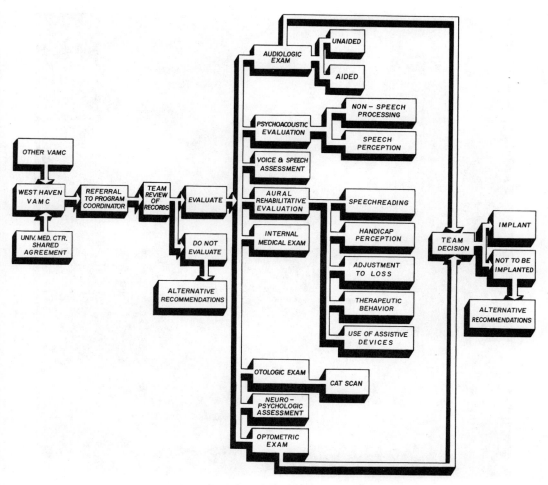

Fig. 1-2. Flow of assessment illustrating involvement of other specialists.

tic team reviews the patient's status and determines the rehabilitative plan to be implemented, whether it should involve further aural rehabilitation with a hearing aid, vibrotactile device, or cochlear implantation.

DEVICES IN USE TODAY—AND CAVEATS

The content of this text assumes that the reader has had graduate level coursework in the technical aspects of hearing aid function and fitting. Such material will not be reviewed here. (For extensive discussion of hearing aid–related topics, the reader is referred to Pollack, 1980; Loavenbruk and Madell, 1981; or Stude-

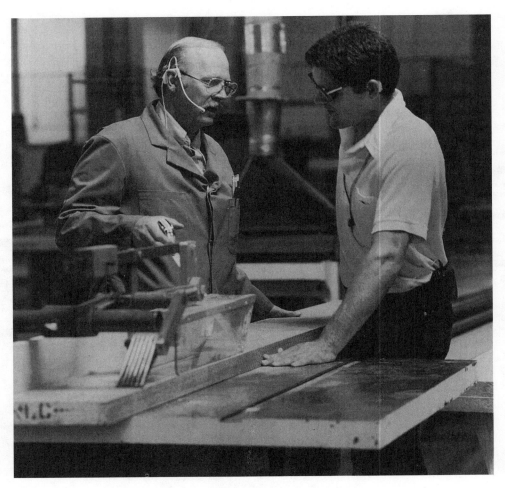

Fig. 1-3. Hearing aid being used in conjunction with an assistive listening device (ALD) in a work setting. *(Courtesy Comtek.)*

baker, Bess, and Beck, 1991.) However, in recent years, a growing trend toward the use of assistive listening devices in conjunction with powerful hearing aids is worthy of note.

A variety of devices may be used to enhance the use of a hearing aid by a severely or profoundly impaired adult. In the past, the use of devices such as auditory trainers was more common in schools for the deaf but was relatively infrequent by adults. Presently, owing to both technologic improvements as well as increasing acknowledgement of the limitations of conventional hearing aids in many listening environments, assistive listening devices are often suggested as a

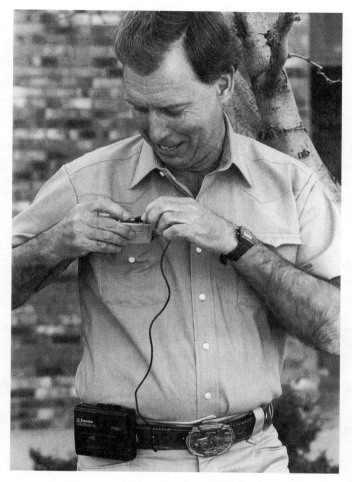

Fig. 1-4. Cochlear implant used with an adult patient. Note use of ALD. *(Courtesy Cochlear Corporation.)*

means for overcoming adverse communicative situations. Many adults with late-onset deafness have been encouraged to use FM auditory trainers, infrared assistive devices, and hardwire arrangements to overcome oft-cited problems associated with meetings in the workplace, large social gatherings, television listening, and the like. (For a full discussion of ALDs, see Vaughn, Lightfoot, and Teter, 1988; Garstecki, 1988.) In this text, the therapeutic situation may require the use of a powerful hearing aid in conjunction with an ALD, as shown in Fig. 1-3.

Cochlear implants are a class of devices that entail surgical implantation of (an) electrode(s) into the cochlea. Implants have also been described in which the placement of the electrode(s) is within the middle ear (i.e., "extracochlear" implants) or within the nervous system (i.e., "cochlear nucleus" implants). At this time in the United States, the most common placement for stimulating electrodes is within the cochlea via the round window. Several texts (Owens and Kessler, 1989; Miller and Spelman, 1990; Cooper, 1991) are resources for background and practical information. In addition, there is a plethora of journal publications regarding the safety and efficacy of implants (Pickett and McFarland, 1985). There are indications in the literature that the effectiveness of implants may allow some users to have limited conversational ability over the telephone (Cohen, Waltzman, and Shapiro, 1989; Dorman, Dove, Jarkin et al., 1991); however, further study is needed. Examples of contemporary cochlear implants, which may also be used in conjunction with ALDs, are illustrated in Figs. 1-4 and 1-5.

Vibrotactile aids have also evolved in complexity of signal processing in the past decade (Proctor, 1984; Reed, Durlach and Braida, 1982; Boothroyd, 1988). Providing a vibratory image of the speech signal, the output transducer(s) can be worn on the hand, wrist, chest, or across the upper back. A number of articles document the effectiveness of vibrotactile aids in adult users (Skinner et al., 1988; Kishon-Rabin, Boothroyd, Eran et al., 1990) as well as in children (Henoch and

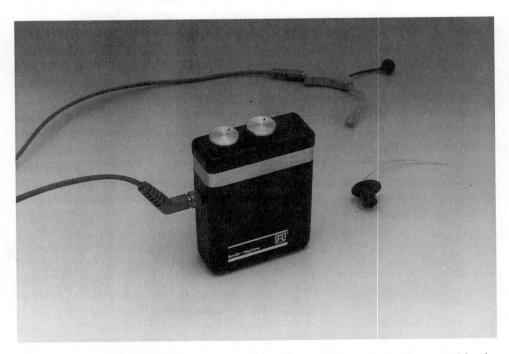

Fig. 1-5. Cochlear implant that can be used with an adult patient. *(Courtesy Richards-Nephew-Smith Corporation.)*

Hunt, 1981; Proctor, 1983). It is possible for an adult user to perform very impressively using a vibrotactile device (Cholewiak and Sherrick, 1986). Further, it has also been suggested that use of a tactile aid may serve as a "bridge" in developing sound responsivity in a candidate who ultimately undergoes cochlear implantation (Miyamoto, Meyers, and Punch, 1987). The reader is referred to Summers (1992) for a comprehensive discussion of the theoretic and practical aspects of tactile aids. An adult wearing a multichannel vibrotactile device is shown in Fig. 1-6.

There are two caveats that must be made here. The first relates to contemporary devices. The reader should note that other devices, such as the Upton eyeglasses (Upton, 1968), were tried with less than general acceptance or success. In fact, devices in use today may soon be eclipsed by later generations, which are more sophisticated in their physical design, speech-processing scheme, or relative effectiveness. It is also true that any rehabilitative plan must take into account the processing constraints inherent in the device the patient uses. Nevertheless, philosophically, we believe that rehabilitative planning will continue to be relevant as improvements in the assistive devices are made available. Many aspects of ther-

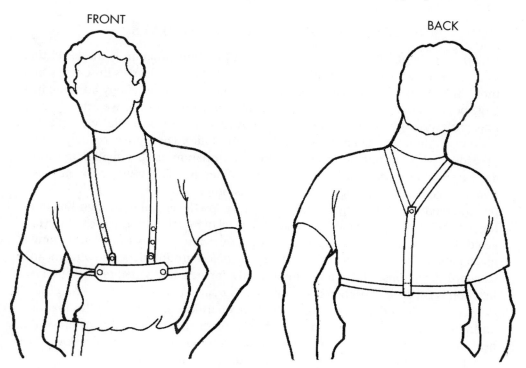

FRONT   BACK

Fig. 1-6. Illustration of an adult using a multichannel vibrotactile aid in an abdominal placement. *(Courtesy Audiological Engineering.)*

apy will remain necessary because the person receiving the device still has needs that must be met.

A second important caveat, sometimes ignored because of the attention paid to various technologic approaches used to solve the communicative problems of the hearing impaired, is recognizing the importance of alternative communication systems, such as the use of American Sign Language (ASL), signed English, or Cued Speech (Cornett, 1967). Such methods may be appropriate for the late-deafened adult, depending on the person's attitude toward such systems, support and participation of significant others, and the availability of a compatible communicative milieu. While it has been our experience that many late-deafened adults will reject any signing method in an almost reflexive manner, we have also seen adults for whom the use of ASL has been a great boon and who have developed many social ties through its use. Therefore, in individual cases, learning ASL should be given consideration in therapeutic planning. We emphasize in this text an aural-oral approach and do not dwell on ASL or sign systems. The interested reader may pursue this topic in some of the excellent sources available (Hoemann, 1978; Siple, 1978; Wilbur, 1979).

OUR APPROACH: RATIONALE FOR MATERIALS

An underlying tenet in the development of the our program is the belief that skills important for communication in fact exist to varying degrees in severely and profoundly hearing impaired individuals. Normal distribution of any attribute in a large population is reflected among the hearing impaired also, so we can expect to find great variation in the extent of any given skill. For example, we have encountered, clinically, all levels of speechreading ability. There are exceedingly poor lipreaders who are unable to obtain much information at all visually, and there are exceptional ones who can communicate fluently using visual cues only. We hypothesize that lipreading ability, as well as other skills we target for rehabilitative intervention, fall along a continuum, from low-level ability to high functioning. Further, since it is possible to assess the level of function for the each of the targeted skills, our therapeutic starting point can be defined. To assist in determining a given patient's level of function, we offer our subject group's data, showing means, standard deviations, and—more importantly for deciding whether the observed function is *low level* (25th percentile or lower), *moderate* (middle 50%), or *high level* (75th percentile and above)—we present the quartile breakpoints. In this manner, an individualized therapy program can be constructed, which aims to move the hearing-impaired patient as far as possible along the continuum for each skill.

Each section of our modular rehabilitation program (Chapters 2 to 5) is organized to include a straightforward description of the rationale, therapy protocol, procedures, suggested stimuli, and criterion measures. Our intent is to highlight why we felt each therapeutic component was needed by the late-deafened patient and to provide hierarchic guidelines for the implementation of communication training. The approaches presented in the following chapters are examples that must be expanded on by individual clinicians and tailored for specific patients.

SUMMARY

The chapters in this text present a graduated approach to each of the following subareas: counselling regarding impact on daily life (Chapter 2), auditory training with reference to training with vibrotactile aids (Chapter 3), speechreading training methods (Chapter 4), and voice and resonance (Chapter 5). Embedded in each of these chapters are implicit measurement procedures that may be new to the reader. We have, therefore, provided resource listings regarding self-help as well as information or materials sources (Chapter 6) and bibliographic citations to permit further guided reading regarding rehabilitative methods in general or our procedures in particular.

In a complex, developing area such as adult aural rehabilitation, it would be unrealistic to suggest that a single text or handbook could provide all the necessary information for designing rehabilitative plans. Our attempt is to make a circumspect step in that direction, offering specific guidelines as well as providing the reference materials to permit talented clinicians in the field to tailor their individualized approaches both to the unique patient and to their own unique therapeutic style.

REFERENCES

Bebout JM: The Americans with Disabilities Act, *Hearing J* 43:11-19, 1991.

Boothroyd A, editor: Auditory and tactile presentation of voice fundamental frequency as a supplement to speech reading, *Ear Hear* 9, 1988.

Cholewiak RW, Sherrick CE: Tracking skill of a deaf person with long-term tactile aid experience: a case study, *J Rehab Res* 23:20-26, 1986.

Clark GM, O'Loughlin BJ, Richards FW et al: The clinical assessment of cochlear implant patients, *J Laryngol Otol* 91:697-708, 1977.

Cohen N, Waltzman S, Shapiro W: Telephone speech comprehension with use of the Nucleus cochlear implant, *Ann Otol Rhinol Laryngol* 9:8-11, 1989.

Committee on Rehabilitative Audiology: Definition of and competencies for aural rehabilitation, *Asha* 26:37-39, 1984.

Cooper H: *Cochlear implants—a practical guide,* San Diego, 1991, Singular Publishing.

Cornett RO: Cued speech, *Am Ann Deaf* 112:3-13, 1967.

Dorman MF, Dove H, Parkin J et al: Telephone use by patients fitted with the Ineraid cochlear implant, *Ear Hear* 12:368-369, 1991.

Eisenberg LS, Maltan AA, Portillo DW et al: Electrical stimulation of the auditory brainstem structure in deafened adults, *J Rehab Res Dev* 24:9-22, 1987.

Espir MLE, Rose FC: *Basic neurology of speech,* Oxford, 1976, Blackwell.

Garstecki D: Considerations in selecting assistive devices for hearing impaired adults, *J Acad Rehab Aud* 21:153-157, 1988.

Goehl H, Kaufman D: Do the effects of adventitious deafness include disordered speech? *J Speech Hear Dis* 49:58-64, 1984.

Henoch M, Hunt S: Application of a vibrotactile aid in improvement of speech in deaf children, *J Acad Rehab Aud* 14:125-140, 1981.

Hoemann HW: *Communicating with deaf people,* Baltimore, 1978, University Park Press.

House WF, Berliner KI: Cochlear implants: progress and perspectives, *Ann Otol Rhinol Laryngol* 91:1-124, 1982.

Kishon-Rabin L, Boothroyd A, Eran O et al: Speechreading enhancement: single versus multichannel tactile transmission of voice fundamentals, Paper presented at the annual convention of the American Speech-Language-Hearing Association, Seattle, November, 1990.

Kline D, Schieber F: Vision and aging. In Birren JE, Schaie KW, editors: *Handbook of the psychology of aging,* ed 2, New York, 1985, Van Nostrand & Reinhold, pp 296-331.

Konigsmark BW, Gorlin RJ: *Genetic and metabolic deafness,* Philadelphia, 1976, WB Saunders.

Leder SB, Spitzer JB: A perceptual evaluation of the speech of adventitiously deaf adult males, *Ear Hear* 11:169-175, 1990.

Leder SB, Spitzer JB, Flevaris-Phillips C et al: Innovative approaches to the selection of cochlear implant candidates, *J Rehab Deaf* 21:27-33, 1987.

Ling D: *Speech and the hearing impaired child: therapy and practice,* Washington, DC, 1976, The Alexander Graham Bell Association for the Deaf.

Loavenbruk AM, Madell JR: *Hearing aid dispensing for audiologists—a guide for clinical service,* New York, 1981, Grune & Stratton.

Luetje CM, Whittaker K, Geier L et al: Feasibility of multichannel human cochlear nucleus stimulation, *Laryngoscope* 102:23-25, 1992.

Mecklenberg DJ, Brimacombe JA: An overview of the Nucleus cochlear implant program, *Semin Hearing* 6:41-51, 1985.

Miller JM, Spelman FA: *Cochlear implants—models of the electrically stimulated ear,* New York, 1990, Springer-Verlag.

Miyamoto RT, Meyers WA, Punch JL: Tactile aids in the evaluation procedure for cochlear implant candidacy, *Hearing Instru* 38:33-37, 1987.

Owens E, Kessler DK: *Cochlear implants in young deaf children,* Boston, 1989, College-Hill.

Pickett J, McFarland W: Auditory implants and tactile aids for the profoundly deaf, *J Speech Hear Res* 28:134-150, 1985.

Pollack MC, editor: *Amplification for the hearing impaired,* New York, 1980, Grune & Stratton.

Proctor A: Tactile aids for the deaf: applications for clinic and classroom, *Folia Phoniatr* 35:3-4; 165, 1983.

Proctor A: Tactile aids for the deaf: a comprehensive bibliography, *Am Ann Deaf* 129:409-416, 1984.

Reed C, Durlach N, Braida L, editors: *Research and tactile communication of speech: a review,* Rockville, MD, 1982, ASHA.

Simmons FB: Some medical, social and psychological considerations in cochlear implants, *Semin Hearing* 6:1-6, 1985.

Siple P: *Understanding language through sign language research,* New York, 1978, Academic Press.

Skinner MW, Binzer SM, Frederickson JM et al: Comparison of benefit from vibrotactile aid and cochlear implant for postlinguistically deaf adults, *Laryngoscope* 98:1092-1099, 1988.

Spitzer JB: A cochlear implant team in a VA setting, *VA Practitioner* 3:50-52, 1986.

Spitzer JB, Perlin R: Optometric findings in the VAMC West Haven Cochlear Implant Trials (unpublished).

Studebaker GA, Bess FH, Beck LB: *The Vanderbilt Hearing Aid Report II,* Parkton, MD, 1991, York Press.

Summers IR, editor: *Tactile aids for the hearing impaired,* London, 1992, Whurr Publishers.

Tyler RS, Type-Murray N, Gantz BJ: Aural rehabilitation, *Otolaryngol Clin N Am* 24:429-445, 1991.

Upton HW: Wearable eyeglass speechreading aid, *Am Ann Deaf* 113:222-229, 1968.

Vaughn G, Lightfoot R, Teter D: Assistive listening devices and systems enhance the lifestyles of hearing impaired persons, *Am J Otol* 9:101-106, 1988.

Wilbur RB: *American Sign Language and sign systems,* Baltimore, 1979, University Park Press.

2

Impact on Daily Living

THERE has been more attention in the deafness literature on the psychologic (Myklebust, 1964) and psychiatric (LeBuffe and LeBuffe, 1979) effects of congenital hearing loss than on such effects associated with severe or profound hearing loss later in life. Similarly, formal study of the social impact of adventitious deafness has been virtually nonexistent.

A pioneering description of the loss of hearing in adulthood was written by Ramsdell (1962) based on accounts of traumatically impaired servicemen returning from combat after World War II. Ramsdell described depressive reactions in deafened adults, whether hearing loss was sudden or gradual. He attributed the soldiers' depression to loss of function at the *primitive level of hearing,* where contact with the auditory background is maintained. Loss of the *symbolic level of audition,* necessary for linguistic communication, and loss of the *signal or warning level* are also likely to result, at least to some degree, with severe or profound late-onset hearing impairment. Thus, without adequate input from sensory aids to maintain a feeling of connectedness to one's surroundings and to provide warning (or more sophisticated) signals about the environment, the adventitiously impaired adult may develop many adverse responses, such as fear, lack of trust, suspiciousness, and loss of self-confidence.

The following case study highlights many of the features of loss of contact with the environment and the psychologic impact of late-onset deafness that Ramsdell described:

CASE STUDY 2.1

M.B. was referred to our cochlear implant program in 1985. The original referral clearly indicated a history of severe depression.

At the time we first met, M.B. was 54 years old. He had been in the service from 1949 to 1952, experiencing heavy noise exposure. Formal audiologic examination in 1955 showed bilateral sensorineural hearing loss of a severe degree on the right side and a mild degree on the left. His psychiatric examination at the time diagnosed conversion reaction as a response to his hearing loss.

Throughout the 1950s and 1960s, he was a consistent hearing aid user. In the late 1960s, he began to experience otitis media in the left (better) ear, limiting his use of a hearing aid on that side. As his hearing deteriorated, he continued to express numerous somatic complaints. In 1973, hearing aids were no longer providing any communication benefit. By 1976, he was considered to be markedly depressed with suicidal tendencies. Formal audiologic testing in 1984 indicated total sensorineural deafness.

The man we met in 1985 was withdrawn and had shown instances of a potentially violent behavior pattern. For example, he was a woodsman and hunter who spent much time cleaning his rifles alone in his basement. On one occasion, his wife began to descend the stairs into the basement, and, because M.B. had not been aware of her approach until he saw her shadow nearing him, he whirled around, pointing the rifle, ready to fire.

Based on this and other incidents, M.B.'s family was fearful and desperate for help. While our examinations indicated that he was a cochlear implant candidate on an auditory basis, his psychiatric history and withdrawn behavior made us wary of implanting him. Instead, we insisted on a 6-month trial with a vibrotactile device and simultaneous reenrollment in counselling with a psychologist from his home area.

When M.B. returned after 6 months, a remarkable change in affect was noted. The use of a vibrotactile aid had increased his awareness of his surroundings. He stated that he did not feel fearful that strangers would "sneak up" on him. He was able to relax and participate more in his family life. (We followed this patient further, as will be described on p. 32.)

NEUROPSYCHOLOGIC FINDINGS IN LATE-DEAFENED ADULTS

A number of authors (Vega, 1977; Miller et al., 1978; Crary et al., 1978; McKenna, 1986) have reported the results of neuropsychologic batteries given adventitiously impaired adults who applied for cochlear implantation. There were two motivations for the reports. First, in the early studies of cochlear implantation, it was necessary to determine if the use of electrical stimulation would result in adverse psychologic effects. Vega (1977), Miller et al. (1978), and Crary et al. (1978) demonstrated the absence of negative consequences by lack of change in intellectual and personality measures.

The second area of interest in recent neuropsychologic studies has been on predicting the outcome of cochlear implantation. McKenna (1986) failed to find a relationship between traditional, standardized tests of psychologic status and cochlear implant success. He emphasized, however, that these measures continued to be important in selection of candidates. In a small sample of single-channel implant users, we reported (Spitzer et al., 1987) that selected measures of a psychologic battery were among the most highly correlated variables to a subjective rating of cochlear implant success. The correlated variables, however, were not consistent from one assessment interval (stimulation, 6-months' post-stimulation, 1-year post-stimulation) to another, a finding that seemed to parallel the results of other investigators.

Recently, Knutson et al. (1991) used a number of standardized measures as well as a test of learning of visual sequential patterns, a visual monitoring task, and a measure of the patient's desire to participate in health care (the Health Opinion Survey). Findings indicated that the latter two measures were significant correlates of audiologic outcomes; in fact these measures were more useful as predictors than the traditional neuropsychologic battery.

In another report, Knutson and his coworkers (1991) described findings regarding measures of depression and loneliness, using subscales of the Minnesota Multiphasic Personality Inventory (MMPI) and other specific scales, the Beck Depression Scale, and the UCLA Loneliness Scale. The study was designed to evaluate the impact of multichannel cochlear implantation on psychologic status over 9- and 18-month time periods. The findings suggested that, after 18 months of implant use, there was a reduction in depression, social anxiety, isolation, and suspiciousness. An interesting, perhaps unexpected, finding was that the latter improvements in psychologic status did not correlate with improved audiologic performance. The study findings suggest that the benefits are, at best, complexly related to standardized measures of auditory performance and that the lack of statistical relationship is likely due in part to the high variability with which implantees can do the current battery's tasks.

In 1984, when we began receiving referrals of profoundly hearing-impaired adults, it was clear that our caseload would be potentially complicated from a psychologic, as well as psychosocial, standpoint. Our referral material described patients who had incurred hearing loss from diverse etiologies—head trauma, electrocution, and disease states resulting in prolonged unconsciousness or coma. We, therefore, had a serious concern that our patients might have an organic basis for maladjustment or might have significant limitations in their ability to learn improved coping strategies or to adjust to new forms of sensory input.

In the selection process for rehabilitation, the measures in our battery (Delaney and Spitzer, in press) yielded important descriptive information (Appendix A). Our subjects were quite variable psychologically. By performing a routine battery, we determined that the potential damage to intellectual function that might have accompanied neurologic trauma was not a significant factor. The routine use of the neuropsychologic battery described in the following section allowed us to demonstrate that the patients in our group were psychologically capable of participating in a rehabilitation program and might potentially profit from the experiences and training we had to offer. While, as in any group of patients, intelligence, motivation, and ability to learn might vary, our results showed that it was not necessary to limit rehabilitation because of any preconceived impact of neurologic trauma.

An additional concern early in our program was that one of our treatments (i.e., the use of electrical stimulation in cochlear implants) had not yet been proved at the time to be harmless in terms of psychologic function. It was, therefore, important for us to establish a baseline for pre-implant functional status and to follow patients at prescribed intervals after surgery. Our findings parallel those of several other cochlear implant teams—implantation had no effect on repeated measures of psychologic state.

METHODS OF ASSESSMENT

If this chapter were concerned only with the assessment of the psychologic well-being of the hearing-impaired person, then the thrust would be toward the need for participation of a psychologist or neuropsychologist in an assessment protocol. The background of such individuals would need to demonstrate sensitivity to the evaluational requirements of adults with minimal hearing or total hearing loss. It is clear that the battery of tests to be applied would necessarily have to be tailored to accurately measure intelligence, emotional/mood status, and personality without contamination of the findings by measures that were prejudicial against the hearing impaired. Such a battery is feasible, and the willingness of psychologists to learn about hearing impairment and reexamine their own methods in light of new understanding of the effects of deafness should not be underestimated.

Table 2-1 presents a summary of some of the psychologic measures that we found useful in evaluating our hearing-impaired program participants. The tests listed are traditional tests in the psychologist's armamentarium. The major deviation from normal procedure concerns the need to present instructions and other cues used in standard administration in written form, as needed, and to eliminate those measurements that rely chiefly on the processing of heard material. In the postlingual adult patient population, in contrast to prelingually hearing impaired, it is appropriate to assess vocabulary and memory for linguistic materials. The use of motoric tests and figural perceptions is also appropriate, especially since age-normative data are available in the literature for comparison.

However, this chapter does not deal solely with the traditional psychologic problems of the severely or profoundly hearing impaired. Our discussion relates to the social and communicative effects of the individual's (mal)adjustment and describes issues that must be raised in order to promote the highest possible degree of communicative success. The principal professional who applies these psychologic insights to improve communication—in combination with information about hearing loss and assistive devices—is the audiologist. Modification of communicative behaviors may be directly approached by either the audiologist or a speech-language pathologist on the team.

TABLE 2-1   Summary of psychologic measures and their purposes

Test	Goal of examination
Finger Tapping	Assesses motor speed and control
Pegboard Test (D, N)	Assesses visual/tactile–motor integration or manual dexterity
Trails Test (A, B)	Assesses visual-motor integration and concentration
Weschler Adult Intelligence Scale— revised	Measure of intelligence using tasks involving verbal and nonverbal abilities
Figural Recall of the Weschler-Memory Scale (Russell adaptation)	Tests visual memory, including immediate recall, delayed recall, and percent of information retained over delay
Controlled Oral Association Test (H-words)	Tests speed of production of a narrowly defined aspect of vocabulary
Boston Naming Test	Tests confrontational naming
Minnesota Multiphasic Personality Inventory	Assesses presence of abnormal symptoms in affective and general personality spheres
Beck Depression Scale	Measures extent of symptoms related to depression

Areas that require additional assessment are perceptions of handicap, communicative behaviors, acceptance of hearing impairment or deafness, perception of stigma, degree and effectiveness of family support, knowledge and action regarding support systems for the severely and profoundly impaired, and knowledge and acquisition of assistive devices. Each of these areas and our findings about previous groups of patients will be presented in the discussion that follows. The attitudinal, communicative effectiveness, and social measures are displayed in Table 2-2.

PERCEPTIONS OF HANDICAP

The difference between the term *impairment* and *handicap* has been discussed a great deal in the audiologic literature. Giolas (1990) characterizes the difference as a distinction between ". . . organic status of the auditory mechanism (hearing impairment) and the effect of that impairment on the communicative, social, and emotional status of the individual (hearing handicap)." For an in depth review of the broader issues concerning hearing handicaps in general, the reader is referred to a comprehensive discussion (e.g., Colodzin et al., 1981, or Giolas, 1983).

Our target population is clearly unique, has a narrower definition of hearing impairment, and, therefore, a narrower range of situations in which their hearing

TABLE 2-2   Summary of tests: attitudinal, communicative effectiveness, and social battery

Test	Goal of examination
Performance Inventory for Profound and Severe Loss (PIPSL)	Assesses a variety of communicative situations and response to hearing difficulty; may also be assessed in an index relative
Beliefs About Deafness Scale (BADS)	Examines preconceived barriers to social interaction that the responder attributes to deafness; may also be assessed in an index relative
Use of ALD Survey	Determines present use of ALDs
Use of Community Resources Survey	Determines knowledge and use of community resources for the deaf and hearing-impaired
Behavioral Observation Record (BOR)	Evaluates patient's communicative performance relative to a list of behaviors

can be expected to support them at all. Therefore, it is not necessary to survey a wide variety of situations and range of possible degrees of handicap suggested by such handicap measures as the Hearing Measurement Scale (Noble and Atherley, 1970), the Denver Scale (Alpiner, 1978), or the Hearing Performance Inventory (Giolas, Owens, Lamb et al., 1979) nor is it necessary to restrict assessment because of age limitations in our targeted patients, as was done in the construction of some scales (e.g., Ventry and Weinstein, 1982).

Knutson and Lansing (1990) found that, using the Communication Profile for the Hearing Impaired (CPHI) (Demorest and Erdman, 1984), scores on the Personal Adjustment subscale fell within a similar range for cochlear implant candidates and other hearing-impaired subjects. When Lansing and Seyfried (1990) followed a group of implantees longitudinally (pre-implant, and 1-, 9- and 18-months' post-implantation), CPHI scores changed immediately post-implantation (i.e., by the 1-month assessment). When the authors evaluated the results in greater detail, three patterns of personal adjustment arose: no change, significant change after 1 month of use, and more gradual change over time.

A scale designed especially for assessing perception of handicap in severely and profoundly impaired persons known as the Performance Inventory for Profound and Severe Loss (PIPSL) was introduced by Owens and Raggio (1988) (Appendix B). Six categories of questions were derived: (1) understanding speech with visual cues, (2) intensity, (3) response to auditory failure, (4) environmental sounds, (5) understanding speech with no visual cues, and (6) personal. The authors suggested using the PIPSL as a counselling tool to determine if a patient was making good use of the present prosthesis. Administration of the scale to a significant other (SO) was also suggested to investigate attitudinal differences between the SO and the hearing-impaired adult.

PRECONCEPTIONS ABOUT DEAFNESS

Numerous preconceptions are harbored by the hearing population that adversely affect the hearing-impaired individual's adjustment to his/her adventitious loss. Attaching a stigma to hearing loss and to the use of hearing aids or other assistive devices often impedes both the deafened adult and his/her family from understanding the individual's unique communication problem and/or from seeking constructive avenues of addressing both the communicative and psychologic needs implied. Several studies of the hearing population's perceptions regarding persons wearing different types of aids indicates that the very act of wearing a hearing aid carries a stigma—the so-called "hearing aid effect" (Blood et al., 1977; Danhauer et al., 1980; Iler et al., 1982).

Becker (1981) described 200 congenitally deaf people over the age of 60, all of whom communicated using American Sign Language (ASL). In this group, the recognition of stigmatization and attempts to cope with negative family attitudes (in the case of hearing parents) were early childhood memories. As adults, they remembered feeling devalued both because of their deafness and their use of ASL or gesture. Deaf identity was acquired early in life and formed the basis of bonding to a social support system in the deaf community.

The late-deafened adult lacks these early experiences and often does not form an identity as a deaf person. Instead, negative societal attitudes toward the deaf and poor communicators may be part of the late-deafened adult's attitudinal make-up, which is brought to the rehabilitative process. On the other hand, some adventitiously impaired adults discuss their interactions with hearing members of society in terms similar to the congenitally hearing impaired. Such phrases as "the hearing don't care about the deaf" and "I don't even try to talk to them (the hearing in a business or social situation)" are frequent in counselling sessions with late-deafened persons.

There is an overwhelming lack of awareness of the availability of support systems for hearing-impaired adults, such as Self-Help for the Hard of Hearing (SHHH) and the Association for the Late-Deafened Adult (ALDA) support group.

Spitzer and Flevaris-Phillips (unpublished) constructed a scale to assess beliefs and preconceptions about the abilities and handicap imposed by profound hearing loss. Based on the work of Needham (1979) in examining similar notions concerning blindness, the Beliefs About Deafness Scale (BADS) examines a variety of beliefs that may interfere with rehabilitation. The 40-question scale is a 5-point response paradigm, ranging from 1 (strongly agree) to 5 (strongly disagree). BADS appears in Appendix C.

BADS was normed using three groups of subjects: late-deafened adults (29), students (30), and rehabilitation professionals (36); the total N = 95. For the total score, it was found that deaf adults were significantly different in their beliefs about deafness from both the student (t = 7.21, p < 0.0001) and professional (t = 3.21, p < 0.01) groups. The mean of the total scores for each group, standard deviations, standard errors of the mean, and 95% confidence intervals appear in Table 2-3.

EXPECTATIONS REGARDING BENEFIT OF REHABILITATION

Often, the late-deafened person and his/her family seek rehabilitation with unrealistic expectations. It is quite common for a patient, newly fit with a powerful hearing aid, to express disappointment that he cannot hear his wife clearly when she is speaking in the next room. The new user of a vibrotactile device may complain that the device is not working because he cannot understand in noisy situations. A cochlear implantee may express dissatisfaction because voices sound "squeaky" and conversation cannot be understood without lipreading. These complaints are derived from unrealistic expectations regarding the benefit of the devices being used. Although we attempt to avert these complaints with thorough informational counselling before and during fitting with new prostheses, there is a lurking desire on the part of the participant for the best possible result, to be the one who obtains a "star performance, as the following paragraph illustrates:"

One patient, W.G., highlighted that lingering, unrealistic expectations are difficult to diminish or extinguish. This very intelligent man responded appropriately in all of our preimplantation counselling sessions regarding the realistic probable outcomes of surgery. Nevertheless, the day before surgery, he came to the audiologist to discuss his feelings about

TABLE 2-3   Results of the standardization of the Beliefs About Deafness Scale (BADS) (N = 95)

Group	N	$\overline{X}$ (SD)	SE	95% Confidence interval
Deaf adults	29	119 (19)	4	111-127
Students	30	139 (11)	2	135-143*
Professionals	36	147 (10)	2	141-143*

*Significantly different from deaf subjects. See text.

the upcoming surgery and revealed that he had constructed a 10-point scale to describe what he thought about the possible outcomes. On his scale, W.G. considered a surgical failure (i.e., hearing nothing) a "0" and normal hearing a "10." He said he thought that he would probably obtain benefit of "about 4 or 5," meaning that he would hear many sounds and communicate better, especially with lipreading. He ended the conversation by saying: "Wouldn't it be nice, though, if I could get a '10'?" Despite his intellectual understanding of the limitations of the process he was about to begin, he still reserved hope for normal hearing.

We attempt to extinguish these unrealistic expectations early in the counselling process. By using a short questionnaire, such as the Cochlear Implant Expectations Questionnaire (Appendix D), we assess the formal information that the patient has absorbed. Review of responses permits a forum for discussion of the affective responses that are commonly observed and begins a process of preparing the patient for the feelings that may be experienced while undergoing various stages of rehabilitation.

Windmill et al. (1987) reported that all of their patients, regardless of eventual success level or cochlear implant used, experienced disappointment in the early stages following stimulation with their device. They observed that "we have found it extremely difficult to convey the possibility of failure, or even of 'average' performance, to candidates. Media sensationalism, implant team members' descriptions of the 'best' results, plus the patient's psychological state cause the candidate to focus on optimal results and to essentially disregard all negative warnings." Similar sentiments of disappointment were voiced by the subjects in a report by Eisenwort et al. (1990).

Teams working with various assistive devices can all provide case studies of persons who report several indicators of auditory benefit in formal tests, but whose disappointment—inability to accept real benefits that differ from expectations—causes them to become non-users of their device. It is fully possible that hidden, unrelenting, unrealistic expectations may be the real basis for non-use of assistive devices rather than failure to obtain benefit.

We have had similar experiences, not only with our cochlear implantees, but also with persons using other assistive devices. Although it appears that vigorous counselling before fitting does not obviate these responses, it is, nevertheless, important to continue to provide such information. It is necessary to make it clear to the patient that reactions to a new device or a newly acquired communication behavior (such as improved assertiveness) are important to discuss. Encouraging discussion of the patient's reaction and those of others to developing communication skills will give the patient an impartial outlet outside the family or work environment and provide opportunities for the professional to counsel and shape these reactions toward constructive ends.

MODIFICATION OF BROAD COMMUNICATIVE BEHAVIOR

There are several behavioral areas that should be examined in order to determine rehabilitative goals for changing broad communicative performance. Such factors as visual attentiveness, asking for information or clarification, receptive use of facial expression and/or gesture, or use of appropriate pragmatics (such as allowing others to speak and waiting for them to finish their utterance before initiating a response) may be amenable to change. A systematic way to examine these behaviors is by the Behavioral Observation Record (BOR) (Appendix E), which can be used as checklist for tracking communicative acts and their frequencies in a given therapy session. The BOR may also be used as a scoring sheet to evaluate videotaped sessions to determine the frequency of behaviors and to look across therapy sessions to attempt to document improvement, as in a single-subject design approach.

One area that is often addressed in aural rehabilitation is development of assertiveness (see the box on p. 29) This area is also an important goal for the late-deafened adult who may have become very passive in communicative situations. Many significant others and clinicians can also attest that the opposite may occur (i.e., a hearing-impaired adult may manipulate conversational partners by loquaciousness; thus, the hearing impaired may manage to exclude the possibility of communicative failure but do not permit themselves to be placed in a receptive mode). Rehabilitation should focus on encouraging appropriate assertiveness and reinforcing the pragmatic give and take of normal conversation.

FAMILY INFORMATION AND SUPPORT

One of the most challenging areas for counselling is eliciting the understanding and support of family members. Their intellectual understanding of the ramifications of severe or profound deafness may be stimulated by informational counselling, along the lines of informational counselling provided directly to the patient. Lack of knowledge of the effects of hearing loss, the nature of ear disease, mechanisms of communication, effectiveness of various assistive devices, and the emotional effects of hearing loss are prevalent among the family members and other significant persons involved with the hearing-impaired adult. The box on p. 30 summarizes counselling areas that are recommended for family counselling sessions.

Thomas and Herbst (1980) reported on the effects of social isolation in a group of London hearing aid users, many of whom were undoubtedly mildly or moderately hearing impaired. In response to a questionnaire, 34% of the hearing-impaired group indicated that "I have fewer friends than most people" or "I have no friends at all (6%)." Forty percent of the hearing-impaired respondents stated

---

BEHAVIORS STRESSED IN ASSERTIVENESS TRAINING

Positive communication behaviors (to be encouraged)
Asking for assistance when something is missed

("I missed the date of the meeting. When will the meeting take place?")

Getting feedback regarding a portion of the utterance

("I know that you were discussing the movie you saw. Was the movie *Raiders of the Lost Heart?*")

Informing others of hearing impairment

("I have a hearing loss. Would you mind facing me directly while we talk?")

Moving seat to advantageous location

(Sit near front of auditorium or away from extraneous noise sources)

Continuing to try to understand

(Maintain eye contact and use communicative repair strategies when there is some breakdown in understanding; ask speaker to rephrase, simplify, elaborate)

Attempting to anticipate the flow of conversation

(While following the flow of a topic, recognize possible divergences or related topics that may become part of the conversation)

Modifying strategy when initial approach is unsuccessful

("I'm sorry, but I still don't understand that name. Would you mind telling me a word it rhymes with?")

Negative behaviors (to be reduced or extinguished)
Demonstrating impatience when there is communicative failure
Demonstrating tension
Demonstrating hostility

---

they found it very difficult to make friends. As an indication of perceived lack of assistance from others, 25% stated that they had no one to turn to for support in day-to-day life, while 20% felt they had only one supportive person. Further, 27% of the hearing-impaired sample said "I get left out of discussions and decision-making at home." We might project that these trends of limited support and feelings of isolation would be further emphasized in a sample of persons with severe or profound hearing loss.

Indeed, when Spitzer, Kessler, and Bromberg (1992) assessed perceptions of quality of life and hearing handicap in a group of individuals undergoing cochlear implantation, their results highlighted the rehabilitative needs of the adventitiously deaf. In their report, 84 veterans and their index relatives participated in a Depart-

---

AREAS OF FAMILY COUNSELLING

Informational counselling

Nature of sound and, specifically, speech signals
Effects of severe-to-profound deafness on communication
Effects of communication deficits on behavior and emotions
Function of relevant assistive devices; limitations
Family systems

Affective or emotional counselling

Attitudes toward hearing loss and the hearing impaired, including family attitudes
    toward hearing loss and the hearing-impaired family member
Promoting successful communication:
    What is realistic to expect with the assistive device?
    What family behavior is viewed as supportive?
    What family behavior is interpreted as destructive?
Roles of family members in communication:
    How will relationships change as rehabilitation proceeds?
    What is successful adjustment to hearing impairment for significant others and
        the hearing-impaired person?

---

ment of Veterans Affairs (VA) cooperative study examining the effects of two types of multichannel and one kind of single-channel cochlear implants. Seven VA medical centers contributed to the data pool. The subjects responded to two questionnaires, the Quality of Life Questionnaire and the Performance Inventory for Profound and Severe Loss (PIPSL), before implantation and at stimulation, 3-months', 1-year, and 2-years' post-implantation. The index relatives responded to a version of the Quality of Life Questionnaire at the same intervals. The findings reflected a statistically significant improvement in lifestyle and reduced handicap perception immediately post-implantation. The latter trend, toward improved perception of quality of life and reduced handicap, continued to the 3-month assessment interval, with changes being maintained through the 2-year period.

When Spitzer et al. (1992) examined responses of their subjects to individual questions about quality of life, some interesting insights were obtained. For questions regarding safety, isolation, and family relationships, the largest percentage did not perceive a change in their abilities, even in the time period from before implantation to stimulation. For example, when asked "To what degree are you concerned about your safety or welfare because of your deafness?", 41% saw no change, whereas 28% felt less safe and 36% more secure.

When index relatives were asked about their perceptions of change in the safety, social comfort, isolation, and family relationships with the same implantees, they also tended to feel that implantation had not changed their situation. The authors considered it possible that both the implantees and their index relatives may have had unrealistic expectations regarding the degree of impact possible with the device and, therefore, did not see some of the positive impact that occurred. Spitzer et al. (1992) also considered it possible that some of the patients were unable to judge their communicative and social progress because of the effects of mild depressive tendencies measured during the candidate selection process.

Feelings of isolation and frustration also affect significant others. Counselling regarding the affective aspects of deafness should begin early in the patient's rehabilitation process. The family's expectations for change derived from rehabilitation must be adjusted to realistic levels and communicative limits must be accepted. Further, any level of success on the patient's part should be recognized and reinforced.

It is also necessary to recognize that the rehabilitative process itself causes a reshifting of family relationships. Often, among families containing a late-deafened adult, there has occurred a power shift in which the hearing-impaired person is removed from communication within and outside the family. A family member, often the spouse, interprets for other family members and/or strangers and "speaks for" the hearing-impaired person. Frequently, the spouse or significant other reports the content of a conversation to the hearing-impaired person only after the entire contact is finished. The hearing-impaired person is left to ask questions following an interaction to which he/she may have been only a peripheral observer although the subject of the exchange. It is a common complaint that, in situations like physician's appointments, the information— possibly of major health or life or death importance— was communicated only to the person accompanying the hearing-impaired adult, and the hearing-impaired individual was excluded from participation, seemingly by agreement or collusion between the other discussants.

Such maladaptive coping strategies result in further isolation for the hearing-impaired adult and removal from many adult responsibilities and roles. The evolution of a dependent, frustrated individual follows.

During the rehabilitation process, a dramatic change in the dependency relationship may result. A person who formerly allowed his/her spouse to speak will no longer do so. A new cochlear implantee may refuse to use sign language or a private means of communication with his/her significant other that previously had been a hallmark of their successful mutual adjustment to deafness in the family.

The following two case studies illustrate the disruption of family relationships that accompanies the rehabilitative process. In both instances, the family was unprepared for the changes in the patient as the rehabilitative process progressed.

CASE STUDY 2.1 (CONTINUED)

M.B. (described earlier in this chapter) had ceased communicating with his family members in most situations. His solitary lifestyle had developed over many years. His wife had become very protective of him. Whenever they went together for appointments, she did all the talking while M.B. did not participate or try to follow the flow of the conversation. When they came to our clinic, Mrs. B. answered all questions in the initial interview, and Mr. B. permitted this activity without comment. Even when questions were repeatedly directed to M.B., Mrs. B. answered for him. Finally, it was necessary to separate the pair to elicit communication from M.B. himself.

M.B. was implanted with a 3M-House single-channel cochlear implant, as described earlier. At the time of stimulation, M.B. began to communicate more actively and showed new interest in lipreading. When he and his spouse returned for a 6-month follow-up, M.B. was more lively and talkative, whereas Mrs. B. was now sullen and withdrawn. She attempted only rarely to interject or speak for M.B., and, when she did, he very forcefully directed her to stop and allow him to speak for himself. When Mrs. B. spoke privately with the interviewer, she explained that she no longer felt needed by her husband. An intensive course of counselling directed at resolving these issues was begun.

CASE STUDY 2.2

G.T. lost his hearing at the age of 24 as a result of renal failure and ototoxicity. He was an excellent lipreader. He and his wife had learned American Sign Language (ASL) and used it for communication between themselves in most situations.

When G.T. and his wife first came to our clinic, we noted that Mrs. T. served as an ASL interpreter for her husband even though he generally followed a conversation well by lipreading. Sometimes she interpreted immediately when there was any problem conveying information between the interviewer and G.T., disallowing an opportunity to develop effective communication between them.

G.T. received a Nucleus cochlear implant in 1987. He and his wife were ecstatic immediately following his implant stimulation, and it was clear that auditory reception was excellent in formal tests and communicative situations. Early in this process, the pair continued to supplement their own interactions with ASL. The rehabilitation team commented neutrally to the couple that, as time progressed, reliance on ASL would be likely to lessen or stop entirely.

At the time of the 3-month follow-up, Mrs. T. was continuing to sign to her husband. He ignored her and sometimes told her directly to stop. She was not perceptive about the situation and said it was hard to break the habit of signing. As her role changed, she began to express her anger toward team members. She became hostile toward the device itself. She expressed annoyance over minor repair issues that had arisen. As time went on, she took on the role of caretaker of the device, intervening whenever there were repair problems. Interestingly, during these times, because the couple had to revert to use of ASL, she had more control and satisfaction.

In both of the cases described, the spouse felt a loss of power and importance as the hearing-impaired person became more independent and experienced communicative success. A reordering of the family structure was taking place. Dominance patterns from which one partner derived satisfaction changed, and new hierachies developed. In both cases described, the hearing spouse's role in the communication process diminished. It became necessary to promote the spouse's continuing support but to attempt to aid development of a new role. Rather than seeing the new relationship as one in which the significant other has lost identity as a caretaker or leader, a more equitable, interactive relationship should be fostered. By discussing the emerging changes in roles and communication style with the family or a close friend, preparation for change and optimal facilitation can be accomplished.

The methods to be used in accomplishing the counselling goals outlined in our program depend, in part, on the severity of the disruption observed. In moderately or severely disrupted situations, family counselling involving an audiologist and psychologist may be required. (In instances in which another, major psychosocial problem exists—such as alcoholism in the deafened adult—specialized resources accessible to the deaf should be sought.) In less dysfunctional families, the audiologist can provide informational and emotional counselling employing a variety of techniques, including role playing, videotaping interactions with subsequent critiquing, and assertiveness training.

ASSISTIVE DEVICES

It is often quite startling that late-deafened adults and their families are unaware of the numerous devices that have been produced to assist the hearing impaired. Devices such as telecaption decoders for television, hearing dogs, and telecommunication devices for the deaf (TDDs) are virtually unknown outside of the deaf or professional (audiologic or deaf educator) communities. Signalling devices, such as flashing lights or vibrotactile alarms, which have application for lesser degrees of hearing impairment as well as for severe or profound loss, are also not generally well known. Often such devices as FM auditory trainers are associated erroneously only with deaf children. Amplifiers for the telephone, however, are somewhat more broadly understood.

Leder et al. (1988) surveyed a group of 25 adventitiously deaf adults regarding their use of assistive devices (i.e., television caption decoders, telecommunication devices for the deaf [TDDs], and visual and tactile alerting devices). At the time of initial interview, a small percentage of subjects used each type of device—ten subjects (40%) used telecaption decoders, four (16%) used TDDs, and three (12%) used alerting devices. A total of 14 subjects (56%) did not use any assistive device at the time of initial interview. In this group, five (20%) of the subjects were eligible to receive devices from the Department of Veterans Affairs and were provided with appropriate units. The authors counselled the other non-users to obtain a variety of assistive devices. When the patients were followed up 1 year later, nine (36%) remained without any type of assistive device. In fact, none of the subjects who had obtained devices had done so at their own expense.

When evaluating the reason for the low rate of use of assistive devices among the adventitiously impaired, it is possible that inadequate information is available to the general public about the devices' existence and applicability. However, after counselling about the need and appropriateness of such devices for our target population, we found the failure to obtain such technologic support a cause for concern. Barriers to obtaining these devices are not always financial, especially when many state agencies provide certain units, such as TDDs, at minimal or no cost. We can only hope that, based on newly implemented legislation, assistive devices will be in broader use in public places, thus increasing awareness and acceptance of assistive devices by and for the deaf.

COMMUNITY RESOURCES

Social withdrawal caused by deafness also results in informational deficits. Knowledge of community agencies that assist the hearing impaired and deaf is sparse among the adventitiously impaired. Fig. 2-1 outlines a variety of agencies or groups that it is likely the adventitiously hearing impaired adult will not be familiar with. State or federal agencies, private organizations, and self-help groups may be totally unknown to the hearing-impaired person and his/her family. Information regarding contacting these organizations is listed in Chapter 6.

STAGING THE REHABILITATION PLAN

Based on the patient's and/or the family's degree of acceptance of the hearing impairment and the extent/quality of their adjustment to the loss, the communicative plan may need to be staged. It may be necessary to wait to activate an aggressive aural rehabilitative program until the psychologic aspects of adjustment are promoted through counselling, possibly by an audiologist and psychologist team. The therapy plan should be developed in a consensual manner, with clinician and hearing-impaired adult (and family, if possible) defining the desired goals, relating them to test findings, and compromising in the direction of attainable objectives. The goals, as we describe in our chapters, are generic, but it is possible to make them more narrow and specific for a given patient's social or employment setting needs.

The following section provides a general therapy plan, which must be modified to accommodate individualized needs for daily living as well as the hearing-

GOVERNMENT RESOURCES   **PRIVATE SECTOR**

Federal level

Department of Veterans Affairs
National Captioning Institute
NIDCD
FDA

State level

Department of Vocational
  Rehabilitation
State Commission for Deaf and
  Hard of Hearing

Self-help groups

ALDA
SHHH
Suzanne Pathy Speak-up Institute
Veterans groups (DAV, VFW,
  AMVETS, VOHI)

Informational sources

AG Bell Association
AAOO
ASHA
Consumers Organization for the
  Hearing Improvement
HEAR Now
National Information
  Center on Deafness
JAN
Lion's Club
NTID
OUT
Sertoma
Tele-Consumer Hotline

Distributors and manufacturers of
assistive devices

Publications for the hearing
impaired

For explanations of abbreviations and further details, see Chapter 6.

Fig. 2-1. Community resources available for late-deafened adults.

impaired person's level of function or capability for understanding. This section begins the process that is then described in subsequent chapters for specialized training in auditory skills, speechreading, and voice conservation. We begin with therapy plans for activities of daily living, as this section contains the information base for understanding one's hearing impairment and response to the loss. This aspect of therapy also increases knowledge of assistive devices and implements action toward making improvements in their use. Such information is necessary and should generally precede the implementation of other aspects of the rehabilitation process. This section also discusses coping and improving adjustment for the patient and significant other(s).

A few general comments regarding the use of our therapy plans are warranted at this point. First, our therapy plans are not structured so that the clinician can complete one objective in a single therapy session. These objectives are an indication of informational targets for the patient and clinician to accomplish and may require several sessions, depending on such factors as patient sophistication regarding deafness and communication skills. Second, it is often necessary to repeatedly return to a goal or objective for review. Therefore, although therapy plans should reflect progress as one proceeds to more advanced objectives, it is still reasonable to expect that review or reinterpretation of information may be needed at various points. Such review is productive as long as the general course of therapy moves toward more advanced objectives and more sophisticated skills and information level. It is often said that good teaching entails repetition of information; solid learning requires reiteration for most people.

There is, also, to a limited extent, some repetition of topics covered in the present chapter in subsequent chapters. For example, we found it necessary to address broad communicative behavior in the present chapter because of its emotional content and ramifications for family counselling and activation of change. We also deemed it appropriate to review and present, in a slightly different manner, the same material in our speechreading therapy section (Chapter 4) because full implementation of communication strategies cannot be discussed without including these issues in the context of use of visual information.

Finally, this chapter's therapy goals should be regarded as an introduction for the patient and family to what rehabilitation is all about. Many hearing-impaired persons have never had the experience of such intensive training and examination of both performance and feelings. Understanding the therapy process is vital to participation and assumption of responsibility by the patient for his/her own success. Subsequent chapters continue the process by working on additional skills and building on an information base established during the early phase of therapy.

THERAPY PLANS: GOALS, OBJECTIVES, AND SUCCESS CRITERIA
I. Development of an Informational Base for Improved Understanding of Deafness

---

A. GOAL: To *understand* hearing impairment and the goals and methods of the rehabilitation process.

 1. **Objective:** To *learn* about hearing loss in general and one's own loss and rehabilitative options. This step begins the process of developing a common working vocabulary about deafness that is necessary for intelligent participation in rehabilitation.

   Procedure: Discuss the following topics, using the patient's own communication characteristics and problems as illustration whenever possible:
   a. Auditory anatomy
   b. Etiologies of hearing loss, and, if known, the patient's own historical background and limitations in medical treatment for sensorineural hearing loss
   c. Measurement of hearing
   d. Introductory information about use of assistive devices for sensory rehabilitation

   Criterion: Patient demonstrates understanding of the preceding concepts; clinician monitors periodically.

   Materials:
   a. Anatomic charts and/or models
   b. Patient's audiogram
   c. Vocabulary list
     (1) Range of normal hearing
     (2) Severe and profound hearing loss
     (3) Sensorineural hearing loss
     (4) Anatomic sites: outer ear, middle ear, inner ear, auditory nerve, auditory centers of the brain
     (5) Speechreading or lipreading
     (6) Gesture
     (7) Context

 2. **Objective:** To *understand* the rehabilitative process.

   Procedure: Describe the general content and time requirements of the rehabilitation plan (i.e., psychosocial counseling, auditory training, voice/speech conservation, speechreading, communication training, and assistive device use). Discuss the commitment that is required for participation in the rehabilitation program. Present the rehabilitation contract and discuss.

Criterion: Patient demonstrates understanding of the preceding concepts; clinician monitors periodically.

Materials:

a. Outline of therapy

b. Rehabilitation contract

B. **GOAL:** To *understand* and *accept* the sensory assistive devices available today.

   1. **Objective:** To *develop* a knowledge base regarding assistive devices.

   Procedure: Discuss benefits and limitations of hearing aids, cochlear implants, and vibrotactile aids. Show videotapes of interviews with patients who have undergone or are in the process of rehabilitation with such devices. Tapes in this category are available from manufacturers and can also be made by individual centers showing their own patients' responses to the program and the devices they are using. Whenever possible, videotapes with open or closed captions should be employed. Provide patients with reading materials concerning the function, benefits, and limitations of the device(s) under discussion. Patient booklets are produced by manufacturers and may also be devised by a rehabilitation group, reflecting their program's philosophy and methods.

   Discuss specific topics with a prospective cochlear implant candidate. The misconception that an implant will eradicate deafness must be eliminated. The concept that the profoundly deaf person will function better but still be subject to many limitations should be presented and discussed at length. *Perception of the cochlear implant user as a hearing-impaired person should be fostered.* Discuss patient concerns about surgical risks and clarify misconceptions. Those surgical issues that remain must be discussed further (in a team meeting or individual appointment) with the team's otolaryngologist.

   Following sessions in which these issues have been discussed, administer the Cochlear Implant Expectations Questionnaire (Appendix D) to both patient and significant other(s). The responses are the basis for ongoing discussion to promote improved understanding and acceptance of the probable limitations in communication with the prospective device.

   Criterion: Patient understands benefits and limitations of prospective device and rehabilitation plan. This is assessed by ongoing discussion.

   Materials:

   a. Videotapes and patient booklets

   b. Cochlear Implant Expectations Questionnaire (Appendix D)

   c. Vocabulary list

(1) Hearing aids (including names of components, such as earmold, earhook, external or audio input, tele-coil, MT switch)

(2) Cochlear implant (including names of components, such as earhook, microphone, speech processor, transmitter, and specific available adapters relevant to devices in the program's use)

(3) Vibrotactile aid (including names of components, such as speech processor, microphone, vibrator/vibrator array)

(4) Aid to lipreading (speechreading)

(5) Single-channel processing

(6) Multi-channel processing

(7) Auditory awareness vs. auditory discrimination

2. **Objective:** To *develop* a knowledge base concerning other assistive devices and, as appropriate, train patients in their use.

Procedure: Assess the patient's current use of assistive devices; such evaluation may be performed using a pen and pencil questionnaire. Provide reading material about devices available for use in conjunction with the patient's hearing aid, implant, or vibrotactile unit.

When a determination has been made about which devices (e.g., an FM auditory trainer) will meet the patient's lifestyle needs, training in the means to use them in various settings should be carried out. Training should include family members, whenever possible, so that they can gain insight into the functional abilities of the patient in important settings.

Criterion: Patient and family decide which assistive devices they will obtain and act on the decision. They demonstrate ability to use the devices, following instructions accurately 90% of the time.

Materials:

a. Measurement scale for evaluation of assistive device needs, such as an ALD Survey (Kaplan et al., 1985)

b. Informational booklet(s), such as A.G. Bell Association's *Signaling and Assistive Devices for Hearing-Impaired People* (see Chapter 6)

c. Videotaped instructional materials including *Assistive Devices: Doorways to Independence* and *Assistive Devices for Hearing-Impaired Persons* (see Chapter 6)

d. Assistive device as selected for demonstration purposes and its written instructional materials

3. **Objective:** To *develop* ability to use a telecommunication device for the deaf (TDD).

Procedure: Encourage use of a telecommunication device for the deaf (TDD). The patient and family should have experience in using a TDD and be able to consider it as a viable alternative to use of spoken communication over the telephone. A TDD may be necessary to contact the Deafness

Center in the event of malfunction of an assistive device; in addition, it is useful for emergency communication. Training with a TDD should take place, even though the patient will also receive device-specific telephone training during his/her auditory training (see Chapter 3). Training should follow these steps:

a. Demonstrate method for coupling TDD to telephone
b. Instruct in use of turn-taking style used in TDD communication; this aspect should include use of typical TDD code (i.e., GA ("go ahead"); SK ("signing off") (Appendix F)
c. Instruct in use of TDD operator
d. Provide guidance in the development of a personal TDD directory
e. Assess acquisition of TDD skills using the appropriate section of the Component Scale for Telecommunication (see Chapter 3).

Criterion: Patient demonstrates ability to use TDD, following instructions accurately 90% of the time.

Materials:

a. Telephone, TDD, and written instructional materials
b. National TDD Directory, printed summary of TDD codes, and component scale for telecommunication

4. **Objective**: To *increase* awareness of community resources for the hearing impaired.

Procedure: Assess patient and family's knowledge concerning the availability of support systems and resources for the hearing impaired in the community. Assessment may be informal, based on directed conversation, or formal, using a questionnaire developed by an individual Deafness Center using the information in Chapter 6 and tailored to the local city and state organizations.

After determining the patient's current involvement in and use of resources for the deaf, suggestions should be formulated as necessary to enhance patient's support network. These suggestions are then discussed.

Criterion: Patient and significant others understand these concepts and follow those suggestions with which they are most comfortable.

Materials:

a. Community Resource Questionnaire (from local Deafness center)
b. Ongoing discussion

II. Development of an Understanding of the Emotional Ramifications of Severe or Profound Hearing Loss and Enhancement of Coping Skills

A. **GOAL:** To *develop* an understanding of the emotional ramifications of hearing loss in general and in one's own life.

1. **Objective:** To *understand* how behavior is affected by late-onset deafness.
   Procedure: Discuss affective domain, stages of mourning for loss of hearing, and arrival at acceptance of long-term status. Discuss how hearing loss can affect family relationships. Define the terms *impairment* and *handicap* and differentiate between them.
   Criterion: Patient and significant others understand these concepts.
   Materials: Discussion.

2. **Objective:** To *develop* self-awareness regarding attitudes about deafness.
   Procedure: Administer the Beliefs About Deafness Scale (BADS)(Appendix C) to patient and significant other(s). Discuss responses, prejudices regarding the hearing impaired, and how such attitudes can adversely affect the rehabilitative process and relationships.
   Criterion: Patient and significant others understand these concepts.
   Materials:
   a. BADS
   b. Discussion

3. **Objective:** To *develop* self-awareness regarding hearing handicap.
   Procedure: Administer the Performance Inventory for Profound and Severe Loss (PIPSL) (Appendix B) to patient and (index relative version) to significant others. Discuss responses, perceptions of how the patient's severe or profound loss affects performance in numerous daily circumstances, and how such perceptions can adversely affect the rehabilitative process and relationships. Discuss how these perceptions may change as the rehabilitative process continues and as adjustment to an assistive device proceeds. PIPSL may be readministered periodically to assess change due to intervention.
   The patient and significant others may benefit from learning how other patients react to their hearing impairment and how some of these reactions may change over time. Viewing videotaped interviews with other patients may become the basis for further discussions of the impact of deafness in various settings, including the home and workplace.
   Depending on the pattern of patient responses to the PIPSL, direct discussion of the degree of isolation depicted may be necessary. If there are indications of significant isolation, reduction of this tendency should become a focus of counseling.
   Criterion: Patient and significant others understand these concepts.
   Materials:
   a. PIPSL
   b. Videotaped interviews
   c. Ongoing discussion

4. **Objective:** To *gain insight* into how results of personality measures and affective status may reflect impact of hearing loss.

Procedure: After consultation with the team psychologist or in a combined session, pertinent results of the psychologic battery should be discussed. In particular, the findings on the Beck Depression Scale may be significant as well as subscales of the MMPI that give insight into long-term depressive tendencies. Clinicians should use their judgment regarding whether it is advisable to include family or significant others in these sessions.

Criterion: Patient and significant others understand these concepts.

Materials:

a. Findings on psychologic battery
b. Ongoing discussion

III. Improvement of Broad Communicative Behavior

A. GOAL: To *improve* broad verbal and nonverbal communication behaviors.

    1. Objective: To *develop* understanding of verbal communicative behaviors and the communicative process.

    Procedure: Review the following terms and concepts:

    a. Receiver
    b. Sender
    c. Coding
    d. Decoding
    e. Message
    f. Influence of environmental factors on intelligibility (i.e., interference)
    g. Communicative intent (e.g., to exert control, to learn new things, to interact socially, to exchange information)
    h. Gist or grasping concepts
    i. Key words
    j. Topic sentences
    k. Benefits of guessing

    Criterion: Patient and significant others understand these concepts.

    Materials: Discussion.

    2. Objective: To *understand* one's own verbal communication behavior.

    Procedure: Discuss aspects of communication, such as linguistic level and style, directness of expression vs. concealing information, use of humor.

    Criterion: Patient and significant others understand these concepts.

    Materials: Discussion (for patients whose hearing permits it, use of audio- or videotaped conversations as basis for analyzing verbal communication).

    3. Objective: To *develop* understanding of one's own communicative behaviors.

    Procedure: Use the Behavioral Observation Record (BOR) (Appendix E) based on videotapes of previous therapy sessions. Discuss the following negative observations:

a. Demonstration of emotional responses to frustration (irritability, dissatisfaction, anger, hostility)
b. Impulsivity in response style
c. Visual inattentiveness
d. Failure to indicate lack of understanding
e. Poor motivation
f. Not expressing self
g. Not sharing conversational responsibility

Discuss reduction of these observed behaviors in favor of more constructive/productive behaviors (e.g., increasing percentage of time the patient is visually attentive to speaker/sender). Discuss how facial expression, body language, gesture, and mannerisms can influence communication. Describe ways in which the latter factors can support or contradict the verbal message, and how patients and families can improve their style. Discuss how contextual cues may reinforce communication. Discuss strategies for using nonverbal cues as effective reinforcement of the verbal message. Role playing may be a useful technique in reinforcing these behaviors.

Discuss with patient and significant others their positive and negative communication experiences. Have patients analyze the basis of a communicative failure. These sessions should be coordinated in time with training in communicative repair (see Chapter 5).

Criterion: Patient and significant others understand these concepts.

Materials: Discussion (videotaped therapy sessions are basis for analyzing nonverbal communication; patients should analyze their own behavior and be given the opportunity to view videotapes made at successive intervals).

4. **Objective**: To *incorporate* the skills of nonverbal communication, assertiveness in group situations.

Procedure: Discuss manner in which a group situation represents a different, often greater, challenge to effective communication than a one-to-one exchange. Discuss effects of:

a. Signal-to-noise ratio, sometimes adverse
b. Other poor acoustic conditions, such as long reverberation times, poor quality public address systems
c. Distance
d. Lighting conditions
e. Shifting/changing speaker
f. Lack of necessary assistive devices in many public meeting places
g. Limited awareness of effects of hearing impairment in the general population

In order to examine specific group situations and environments in which the patient has difficulty, it may be necessary for a team member to accompany the patient and/or family member to the location to attempt problem-solving. For example, if the patient describes communicative failures in the workplace, at meetings, or in detecting an audio page, the team member may discuss methods of combining use of assistive devices with other newly learned behaviors to improve the situation. Having observed the challenging circumstances, the team member may attempt role playing to simulate the difficult situation and stimulate application of new skills. Role playing of other social situations with family members as participants may be productive.

Criterion: Patient and significant others understand these concepts.

Materials:

a. Discussion
b. Videotapes
c. Role-playing props

5. **Objective:** To *increase* appropriate assertive behavior.

   Procedure: Differentiate between assertiveness and aggressiveness. Describe various assertive behaviors that can affect interactions positively (see box on p. 29.)

   View videotape, *I Can See What You're Saying* (see Chapter 6). Discuss which assertive behaviors were portrayed. Role play situations that the patient regards as difficult (e.g., conversation at the dinner table or restaurant, supermarket shopping, asking directions).

   Criterion: Patient and significant others understand these concepts.

   Materials:

   a. Discussion
   b. Videotapes
   c. Role-playing props
   d. Bill of Rights for Listeners or Talkers (Vaughn, 1986) (Appendix G)

REFERENCES

Alpiner JG: Evaluation of communication function. In *Handbook of rehabilitative audiology*, Baltimore, 1978, Williams & Wilkins, pp 30-66.

Becker G: Coping with stigma: lifelong adaptation of deaf people, *Soc Sci Med* 15(B):21-24, 1981.

Blood GW, Blood IM, Danhauer JL: The hearing aid effect, *Hear Instru* 28:12, 1977.

Colodzin L, Del Polito G, Dickman D et al: ASHA Task Force on the Definition of Hearing Handicap, *Asha* 23:293-297, 1981.

Crary WG, Berliner KI, Wexler M et al: Cochlear implants: a psychological perspective, *J Otolaryngol Soc Aust* 4:201-203, 1978.

Danhauer JL, Blood GW, Blood IM et al: Professional and lay observers' impressions of preschoolers wearing hearing aids, *J Speech Hear Dis* 45:64-71, 1980.

Delaney R, Spitzer JB: Neuropsychological profiles in adventitiously deaf candidates for cochlear implantation (submitted for publication).

Demorest ME, Erdman BE: Psychometric principles in the selection, interpretation, and evaluation of communication self-assessment inventories, *J Speech Hear Dir* 49:226-240, 1984.

Eisenwort B, Kropiunigg U, Burian K: Das Cochlearimplantat und seine psychosozialen Auswirkungen bei 36 Patieten, *Folia Phoniatr* 42:71-76, 1990.

Giolas TG: The self-assessment approach in audiology: state of the art, *Audiology* 3:157-171, 1983.

Giolas TG: "The measurement of hearing handicap" revisited: a 20-year perspective, *Ear Hear* 11(suppl):2S-5S, 1990.

Giolas TG, Owens E, Lamb SH et al: Hearing Performance Inventory, *J Speech Hear Dis* 44:169-195, 1979.

Goodglass H, Kaplan E: *The Boston Naming Test,* Philadelphia, 1983, Lea & Febiger.

Iler KI, Danhauer JL, Mulac A: Peer perceptions of geriatrics wearing hearing aids, *J Speech Hear Dis* 47:433-438, 1982.

Kaplan H, Scott SJ, Garretson C: *Speechreading: a way to improve understanding,* Washington, DC, 1985, Gallaudet College Press.

Knutson JF, Hinrichs JV, Tyler RS et al: Psychological predictors of audiological outcomes of multichannel cochlear implants: preliminary findings, *Ann Otol Rhinol Laryngol* 100:817-822, 1991.

Knutson JF, Lansing CR: The relationship between communication problems and psychological difficulties in persons with profound acquired hearing loss, *J Speech Hear Dis* 55:656-664, 1990.

Lansing CR, Seyfried DN: Longitudinal changes in personal adjustment to hearing loss in adult cochlear implant users, *J Acad Rehab Audiol* 13:63-77, 1990.

Lebuffe FP, Lebuffe LA: Psychiatric aspects of deafness, *Primary Care* 6:295-310, 1979.

Leder S, Spitzer J, Richardson F et al: Sensory rehabilitation of the adventitiously deafened: use of assistive communication and alerting devices, *Volta Rev* 90:19-24, 1988.

Lewis RF, Rennick PM: *Manual for the repeatable cognitive-perceptual-motor battery,* Gross Point Mich, 1979, Axon.

McKenna L: The psychological assessment of cochlear implant patients, *Brit J Audiol* 20:29-34, 1986.

Miller L, Duvall S, Berliner K et al: Cochlear implants: a psychosocial perspective, *J Otolaryngol Soc Aust* 4:201-203, 1978.

Myklebust HR: *Psychology of deafness—sensory deprivation, learning and adjustment,* ed 2, New York, 1964, Grune & Stratton.

Needham WE, Ehmer MN: Irrational thinking and adjustment to loss of vision, *J Vis Impair Blindness* 74:57-61, 1979.

Noble WG, Atherley GRC: The Hearing Measurement Scale: a questionnaire for the assessment of auditory disability, *J Aud Res* 10:229-250, 1970.

Owens E, Raggio MW: Performance Inventory for Profound and Severe Loss (PIPSL), *J Speech Hear Dis* 53:42-57, 1988.

Ramsdell PA: The psychology of the hard-of-hearing and the deafened adult. In Davis H, Silverman SR, editors: *Hearing and deafness,* New York, 1962, Holt, Rinehart, & Winston.

Russell EA: A multiple scoring method for the assessment of complex memory functions, *J Consult Clin Psychol* 43:800-809, 1975.

Russell E, Neuringer L, Goldstein G: *Assessment of brain damage,* New York, 1970, Wiley-Interscience.

Spitzer JB, Flevaris-Phillips CA: The Beliefs About Deafness Scale (BADS) (unpublished study).

Spitzer JB, Kessler MA, Bromberg B: Longitudinal findings in quality of life and perception of handicap following cochlear implantation, *Semin Hear* 13:260-270, 1992.

Spitzer JB, Leder SB, Flevaris-Phillips CA et al: Correlates of cochlear implant success, *Asha* 29:159, 1987.

Thomas A, Herbst KG: Social and psychological implications of acquired deafness for adults of employment age, *Brit J Audiol* 14:76-85, 1980.

Vaughn GR: Bill of rights for listeners and talkers, *Hear Instru* 37:8, 1986.

Vega A: Present neuropsychological status of subjects implanted with auditory prostheses, *Ann Otol Rhinol Laryngol* 86:57-60, 1977.

Ventry IM, Weinstein BE: Self assessment of hearing handicap: a new tool, *Ear Hear* 3:128-134, 1982.

Windmill IM, Martinez SA, Nolph MB et al: The downside of cochlear implants, *Hear J* 40:18-22, 1987.

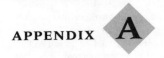

Neuropsychologic Findings

Psychologic characteristics of an adventitiously impaired sample (N = 32)[1]:—means and standard deviations and cut-off scores for abnormal function[2]

Measure	Mean (SD)	Cut-off Score for Abnormal Performance
Intelligence measures		
WAIS-R (Verbal)*	96.11 (13.82)	Below 70[a]
WAIS-R (Performance)*	98.00 (14.31)	
WAIS-R (Full Scale)*	96.68 (13.74)	
Visual/motor integration		
Finger Tapping (D)	50.97 (7.28)	Below 50[b]
Pegboard Test (D)	88.00† (33.94)	Above 66
Trails Test (A)	39.97 (18.78)	Above 33
Visual memory		
Weschler Memory Scale (Immediate Recall)	8.09 (3.36)†	Below 9[c]
Weschler Memory Scale (Delayed Recall)	6.79 (3.79)†	Below 6
Weschler Memory (Visual) percent retained (Russell adaptation)	75.88 (24.96)†	Below 84
Language fluency		
Controlled Oral Association Test (H-words)	15.41 (5.15)	Below 16[b]
Boston Naming Test	53.29 (4.90)	Below 49[d]

(Continued.)

Measure	Mean (SD)	Cut-off Score for Abnormal Performance
Tests of psychopathology (selected)		
Minnesota Multiphasic Personality Inventory—subscales‡		
L	54.41 (10.53)	Above 70
F	59.45 (6.90)	Above 70
K	53.27 (9.23)	Above 70
1	61.82 (15.76)	Above 70
2	64.73 (14.14)†	Above 70
3	59.82 (13.31)	Above 70
4	60.41 (14.94)	Above 70
5	57.23 (8.95)	Above 70
6	57.41 (8.94)	Above 70
7	59.09 (11.35)	Above 70
8	63.14 (13.57)	Above 70
9	58.55 (10.80)	Above 70
10	56.82 (8.12)	Above 70

*Weschler Adult Intelligence Scale—Revised.
†Exceeded age-adjusted normative values.
‡N = 22 for MMPI only.
[1]From Delaney and Spitzer (in press).
[2]Cut-off scores are from a variety of sources:
  [a]Unless otherwise noted, norms are from Russell Neuringer, and Goldstein (1970).
  [b]Lafayette Clinic Norms, Lewis and Rennick (1979).
  [c]Russell (1975).
  [d]Goodglass and Kaplan (1983).

PERFORMANCE INVENTORY FOR PROFOUND AND SEVERE LOSS (PIPSL)*

1. You are at a fairly noisy restaurant talking face-to-face with a male friend or family member. Can you understand what he is saying?

2. Are you able to hear the dial tone on a telephone?

3. When you have difficulty understanding a person with a pipe or toothpick or similar object in his/her mouth, do you ask him/her to remove the object?

4. Can you identify the sound of an orchestra playing on a radio or TV when you have no visual or other cues?

5. Can you understand speech on the radio?

6. Does your hearing loss tend to lower your self-confidence?

7. You are talking to a woman sitting in a ticket or information booth and the surroundings are fairly noisy. She is giving directions or information. Can you understand what she is saying?

8. A man is talking no more than 6 feet away from you. Would you be aware that he is talking if you could not see his face?

9. When you have difficulty understanding a person who speaks rapidly, do you ask him/her to speak more slowly?

10. Can you identify the sound of laughter if you cannot see the person laughing?

11. You hear a stranger talking to another person in a fairly quiet room. Can you understand what she is saying at those times when, for some reason, you *cannot* watch her lip movements?

---

*6 Always, 5 Practically always, 4 Frequently, 3 About half the time, 2 Occasionally, 1 Never, 0 Does not apply. Score sheet for inventory appears on p. 53.

12. Are family members impatient in communicating with you?

13. You are with two or three friends or family members sitting around a table talking. Sometimes people interrupt each other. When you are aware of the general topic, can you follow what is being said?

14. When others are listening to speech on TV or radio, is it loud enough for you?

15. You are talking with five or six friends or family members. When you miss something that you think might be important, do you keep trying by some means to understand?

16. You are in a fairly quiet place and you hear the voice of someone you don't know. Can you tell whether it's a man or woman if there are no visual or other cues?

17. You are with a female friend or family member who is talking to another person in a fairly quiet room. Can you understand what she is saying at those times when, for some reason, you *cannot* watch her lip movements?

18. Do you feel a strong emotion such as anger, sadness, or frustration when you feel left out of an interesting discussion because of your hearing loss?

19. You are at a fairly quiet restaurant talking face-to-face with a female friend or family member. Can you understand what she is saying?

20. You are sitting in a room and people are talking in another room. Can you hear the sound of their voices?

21. You are in a conversation with another person and you have already interrupted twice to understand a word or phrase that you think might be important. Do you keep trying, by some means, to understand this word or phrase?

22. Can you identify the sound of your name when someone calls you from behind?

23. Can you understand what a woman is saying on the telephone?

24. Do you feel that your hearing loss is a social handicap?

25. You are watching a movie or drama on TV. Can you follow the story when there are no captions?

26. Do you feel that children (6 to 10 years old) speak loudly enough for you?

27. You are seated with five or six friends or family members around a table or in a living room. Often two persons are talking at once and one person frequently interrupts another. If the speaker turns away and you miss something that you think might be important, do you, by some means, remind the speaker that s/he must be facing toward you so that you can use lipreading?

28. You hear a friend or family member talking in a fairly quiet place. Can you identify who it is if there are no visual or other cues?

29. You are with a male friend or family member who is talking to another person in a fairly noisy room. Can you understand what he is saying at those times when, for some reason, you *cannot* watch his lip movements?

30. Does your hearing loss make you feel tense?

31. You are talking with a male friend or family member face-to-face in a fairly noisy room. Can you understand what he is saying?

32. There is a telephone in the room where you are sitting. If the phone rings, can you hear it without other cues such as a flashing light?

33. You are talking with a friend or family member. When you miss something that you think might be important, do you keep trying by some means to understand?

34. Can you identify the sound of a human voice if you have no visual or other cues that someone is talking?

35. If you *cannot* see a speaker's face, can you understand that person when s/he makes it a point to speak more slowly and distinctly?

36. Are persons with normal hearing, other than friends or family members, uncomfortable when communicating with you?

37. You are with two or three friends or family members sitting around a table talking. People sometimes interrupt each other. If you are not immediately aware of the general topic do you eventually become aware of it?

38. A woman is talking no more than 6 feet away from you. Would you be aware that she is talking if you could not see her face?

39. You are having difficulty communicating with someone and you are not certain s/he knows you have a severe hearing loss. Do you tell him/her?

40. Can you identify the sound of coughing if you cannot see the person?

41. You hear a child (6 to 10 years old) talking to another person in a fairly quiet room. Can you understand what s/he is saying at those times when, for some reason, you *cannot* watch his/her lip movements?

42. Does your hearing loss tend to make you impatient?

43. You are riding in the front seat of an automobile with a friend who is driving. If he/she is talking can you understand what is being said?

44. When an announcement is given over the public address system in a bus station or airport, are you aware of the sound?

45. When you have difficulty understanding a person because he is holding his hand in front of his mouth, do you ask him to lower the hand?

46. Can you identify the sound of a siren if there are no other cues such as a flashing light?

47. You are with a male friend or family member who is talking to another person in a fairly quiet room. Can you understand what he is saying at those times when, for some reason, you *cannot* watch his lip movements?

48. Do you feel others cannot understand what it is to have a hearing problem?

49. You are at a fairly noisy restaurant. Can you understand the waiter or waitress when you can see his/her face?

50. Are female voices loud enough for you in face-to-face conversations?

51. You are talking with five or six strangers. When you miss something that you think might be important, do you let the person talking know, at least once, that you have a hearing problem?

52. You are talking with a male friend or family member face-to-face in a fairly quiet room. Can you understand what he is saying?

53. You are at home. Can you hear the doorbell ring when it is located in the same room and there are no other cues such as a flashing light?

54. You are playing cards, Monopoly, or some similar game with two or three friends or family members. Can you follow enough of the player interaction to play successfully?

55. You are talking with a male stranger face-to-face in a fairly noisy room. Can you understand what he is saying?

56. You are in a church or auditorium attending a lecture or sermon. Can you understand what is being said when you have a good view of the speaker's face?

57. You are with five or six friends or family members sitting around a table talking. Sometimes people interrupt each other. When you are aware of the general topic, can you follow what is being said?

58. You are talking with a female friend or family member face-to-face in a fairly noisy room. Can you understand what she is saying?

59. How often can you do something about poor lighting that impairs your lip-reading ability?

60. Can you prevent distractions from interfering with your lipreading?

61. You are talking with a friend or family member. When you miss something that you think might be important, do you avoid pretending that you have understood?

62. You are talking with a friend or family member and you understand only a portion of what was said. Do you feedback that portion to the speaker so that s/he can fill in the part you did not understand?

63. If there is one person you can lipread better than anyone else, how often can you understand this person when you can see his/her face?

64. When you are having difficulty conversing with another person, does it help when a friend or family member acts as a go-between?

65. A person is using meaningful gestures while talking with you face-to-face. Are these gestures useful to you in understanding what the person is saying?

66. When you are talking, are you confident that the loudness of your voice is appropriate for the situation?

67. When you are shopping alone, can you communicate with clerks successfully in obtaining what you want?

68. If your hearing is such that you can hear a voice on the telephone but cannot understand what is being said, do you ask the other person to use a code— like "yes", "no-no", "I don't know"— so that you can ask specific questions and understand the answers by counting the syllables?

69. Do you feel generally as safe as others regarding common safety considerations?

70. You are talking with a co-worker face-to-face while working in a fairly quiet area. Can you understand what s/he is saying?

71. You are talking with your employer and you understand only a portion of something that was said. Do you feedback that portion so that s/he can fill in the part that you did not understand?

72. Can you continue learning things connected with your job despite your hearing loss?

73. You are talking with a co-worker on the job. When you miss something that you think might be important, do you avoid pretending that you have understood?

74. You are talking with a co-worker face-to-face while working in a fairly noisy area. Can you understand what s/he is saying?

From Owens E, Raggio MW: *J Speech Hear Dis* 53:42-57, 1988.

Always	Practically always	Frequently	About half the time	Occasionally	Almost never	Never	Does not apply
☐	☐	☐	☐	☐	☐	☐	☐
6	5	4	3	2	1	0	

Score Sheet and Profile

Name _____

Date _____

Amplification _____

Note: For quick tabulation from the answer sheet, proceed from left to right across columns by row.

USV(15)	INT(10)	RAF(9)	ES(8)	USNV(8)	PER(8)*	GEN(15)
1 ____	2 ____	3 ____	4 ____	5 ____	6 ____	59 ____
7	8 ____	9 ____	10 ____	11 ____	12 ____	60 ____
13 ____	14 ____	15 ____	16 ____	17 ____	18 ____	61 ____
19 ____	20 ____	21 ____	22 ____	23 ____	24 ____	62 ____
25 ____	26 ____	27 ____	28 ____	29 ____	30 ____	63 ____
31 ____	32 ____	33 ____	34 ____	35 ____	36 ____	64 ____
37 ____	38 ____	39 ____	40 ____	41 ____	42 ____	65 ____
43 ____	44 ____	45 ____	46 ____	47 ____	48 ____	66 ____
49 ____	50 ____	51 ____				67 ____
52 ____	53 ____					68 ____
54 ____						69 ____
55 ____						†70 ____
56 ____						†71 ____
57 ____						†72 ____
58 ____						†73 ____
						†74 ____
SUM ____	____	____	____	____	____	
#ATT. ____	____	____	____	____	____	
MEAN ____	____	____	____	____	____	

	USV	INT	RAF	ES	USNV	PER	
6.0							6.0
5.5							5.5
5.0							5.0
4.5							4.5
4.0							4.0
3.5							3.5
3.0							3.0
2.5							2.5
2.0							2.0
1.5							1.5
1.0							1.0
0.5							0.5
0.0							0.0

USV = Understanding Speech with Visual Cues
INT = Intensity
RAF = Response to Auditory Failure
ES = Environmental Sounds
USNV = Understanding Speech with No Visual Cues
PER = Personal

*Numeric responses must be reversed before the scoring process: 6 becomes 0 and 0 becomes 6; 5 becomes 1 and 1 becomes 5; 4 becomes 2 and 2 becomes 4.
†Occupational.

BELIEFS ABOUT DEAFNESS SCALE (BADS)

	Strongly Agree	Agree	Neutral	Disagree	Strongly Disagree
1. It is impossible for hearing people to know what it is like to be deaf.	1	2	3	4	5
2. If a deaf person had hearing, he/she would most certainly have a happy life.	1	2	3	4	5
3. Hearing people generally dislike being with deaf people because they are deaf.	1	2	3	4	5
4. Deaf people have to depend on hearing people to do most of the things they did for themselves.	1	2	3	4	5
5. Previous ambitions have to be drastically curtailed following the onset of deafness.	1	2	3	4	5
6. Deafness is a punishment for people who have failed to do what they should.	1	2	3	4	5

	Strongly Agree	Agree	Neutral	Disagree	Strongly Disagree
7. Miraculous cures of deafness are possible.	1	2	3	4	5
8. Deaf people should not expect to be treated like hearing people because they are deaf.	1	2	3	4	5
9. Deaf people should get more help than they usually receive.	1	2	3	4	5
10. It would probably be easier for deaf people to live with spouses who are deaf too.	1	2	3	4	5
11. Deaf people could do everything for themselves if they had enough scientific electronic equipment or aids.	1	2	3	4	5
12. Being deaf is better than hearing all the ugliness in the world.	1	2	3	4	5
13. Being deaf is no handicap.	1	2	3	4	5
14. If a deaf person were married, deafness would be less of a problem.	1	2	3	4	5
15. If a deaf person were single, deafness would be less of a problem.	1	2	3	4	5
16. Being deaf is worse than being blind, diabetic, or wheelchair bound.	1	2	3	4	5

	Strongly Agree	Agree	Neutral	Disagree	Strongly Disagree
	1	2	3	4	5
17. Deaf people get upset when they have to ask for help.	1	2	3	4	5
18. Deaf people get upset when people refuse to help them.	1	2	3	4	5
19. Given the chance, most deaf people could be as successful as either Thomas Edison or Patricia O'Neal.	1	2	3	4	5
20. People should provide substantial financial support for the deaf.	1	2	3	4	5
21. Lipreading is of little use to the deaf.	1	2	3	4	5
22. Deaf people don't need to know how to cook or clean house for themselves.	1	2	3	4	5
23. Those who are deaf should teach others what deafness is like.	1	2	3	4	5
24. When a person becomes deaf, hearing friends don't understand him/her as they did before.	1	2	3	4	5
25. Most deaf people are ashamed to go out in public because they are deaf.	1	2	3	4	5
26. A deaf person who accepts his/her deafness can do anything he/she wants to.	1	2	3	4	5

	Strongly Agree	Agree	Neutral	Disagree	Strongly Disagree
27. With the right medi-cine deafness can be cured.	1	2	3	4	5
28. Life is meaningless for the deaf person who can't work.	1	2	3	4	5
29. Only the deaf can un-derstand the deaf.	1	2	3	4	5
30. A new life must be started after a person becomes deaf.	1	2	3	4	5
31. Many deaf people are unable to hear any-thing at all.	1	2	3	4	5
32. Losing one's hearing means losing one's self.	1	2	3	4	5
33. Deafness causes most of the problems that an individual experi-ences at home, at school, and at work.	1	2	3	4	5
34. Deaf people are more discriminated against than other minority groups.	1	2	3	4	5
35. Deafness is less of a problem for those who are married than for those who are sin-gle.	1	2	3	4	5
36. Loss of hearing makes it harder to find hap-piness.	1	2	3	4	5
37. Deafness breaks up marriages.	1	2	3	4	5

	Strongly Agree	Agree	Neutral	Disagree	Strongly Disagree
38. Deaf people must realize that they can't expect the same rights as other people.	1	2	3	4	5
39. Deafness is merely an inconvenience.	1	2	3	4	5
40. A person's worth is a function of physical intactness.	1	2	3	4	5

COCHLEAR IMPLANT EXPECTATIONS QUESTIONNAIRE

Please answer each question to the best of your knowledge.

1. Can the cochlear implant restore normal hearing?

2. Will the cochlear implant allow you to understand speech?

3. What do you believe the cochlear implant will do for you?

4. What would you like to be able to hear?

5. Is training necessary in conjunction with the cochlear implant? If your answer is yes, what does the training entail?

6. Are you willing to keep a diary of listening experiences and practice listening and speech reading exercises if you are the recipient of an implant or become part of our evaluation program?

BEHAVIORAL OBSERVATION RECORD (BOR)

Instructions to observer: Please note the number of occurrences of each of the following behaviors during the session:

Negative Behaviors	Frequency	Positive Behaviors	Frequency
Expresses irritability	_____	Expresses relaxed attitude	_____
Expresses dissatisfaction	_____	Expresses satisfaction	_____
Responds/shows anger	_____	Responds/shows positive attitude	_____
Shows frustration	_____	Shows self-assurance	_____
Fails to modify actions on request	_____	Modifies actions on request	_____
Acts impulsively to partial stimuli	_____	Waits to hear/see complete stimuli	_____
Shows inattention on auditory basis	_____	Shows attention on auditory basis	_____
Shows inattention on visual basis	_____	Shows attention on visual basis	_____
Shows hostility	_____	Shows cooperative attitude	_____
Does not give indication on failing to comprehend	_____	Gives indication on failing to comprehend	_____
Shows lack of motivation	_____	Shows motivation	_____
Is taciturn	_____	Expresses self	_____
Allows another to take control of conversation	_____	Shares control of conversation	_____
Monopolizes conversation	_____	Allows give-and-take in conversation	_____
Voice breaks/too low	_____	Modulates voice	_____
Produces misarticulations	_____	Produces accurate articulations	_____

Veterans Administration Medical Center. 950 Campbell Avenue, West Haven, Conn.

Terminology Used with a Telecommunication Device for the Deaf (TDD)

Terminology used with a telecommunication device for the deaf (TDD)

Common Term	Meaning
GA	Go ahead
SK	Send-kill; end of communication
HD	Hold
TDD	Telecommunication device for the deaf (TDD) (text telephone)
TTY	Teletypewriter; older device than the TDD; this term continues to be used by many people interchangeably with TDD
CD	Could
U	You
UR	You are; your
PLS	Please
Q	Indicates a question
R	Are
OPR	Operator
NBR	Number
CUL	See you later
OIC	Oh, I see
MTG	Meeting

APPENDIX **G**

Bill of Rights for Listeners
or Talkers

Bill of rights for listeners or talkers

Personal Rights	Communication Rights
Entitlement to quality health care	In receiving areas, hospitals, nursing homes, outpatient waiting rooms, reception areas, physicians' offices, and rehabilitation settings
Opportunity for equal employment	During job interviews, in telephone usage, and in employment in the professions, offices, industry, and fine arts
Protection of legal rights	Through availability of ALDs in police stations, courtrooms, and jails
Admittance to legislative and diplomatic action	In town meetings, state legislatures, Congress, and international organizations
Participation in business activities	In negotiations, conferences, meetings and contacts with bank tellers, telephone operators, receptionists, and managers
Access to protection	By fire departments, emergency services, and police
Assurance of safety	In industry, home, public and private buildings, hotels, airports, and places of public assembly
Recognition of dignity as listener and talker	In interpersonal communication with family and friends in restaurants, social gatherings, automobiles, and over the telephone
Freedom of religion	In worship services, counseling sessions, and confessionals
Opportunity to travel	Through accessibility to translation services, lectures by guides, recorded information at historic sites, and verbal exchange with group members
Understanding of information	Through graphic displays or ALDs in conjunction with public address and signaling systems, public telephones, and radio and television

Personal Rights	Communication Rights
Obtainment of basic and continuing education	Through amplication systems, through tutoring, teleconferencing, and video and audio recordings
Appreciation of entertainment	In concert halls, theaters, and movies
Participation in recreational activities	In indoor and outdoor games, active and spectator sports, and table and group games

From Vaughn GR: *Hear Instru* 37:8, 1986.

CHAPTER 3

Speech Perception Training: Auditory, Vibrotactile, and Electrical Stimulation— Methods and Samples

PROTOCOL outlined in this chapter is designed to assist the late-deafened adult improve speech perception performance. It is based on the assumption that fitting the individual with an assistive listening device is only the beginning of rehabilitation. A more difficult aspect of the process is to provide the hearing-impaired person with effective skills to make use of the speech perception cues made available by the particular assistive device being worn (e.g., hearing aid, vibrotactile unit, or cochlear implant). This process is traditionally referred to as *auditory training*.

Auditory training is defined as the "process whereby the aurally handicapped person learns to take advantage of all acoustic cues available" (Nicolosi, Harryman, and Kresheck, 1978). Although auditory training programs come in a variety of forms, they are typically rooted in one of two methods: (1) the *analytic* method, which teaches recognition of speech sounds in isolation, then in words, sentences, and phrases, or (2) the *synthetic* method, which teaches recognition of the meaning of whole paragraphs before breaking them into sentences, words, and sounds (Nicolosi et al., 1978). Most current programs used with the profoundly hearing-impaired adult include a combination of both approaches: which is emphasized is based on the individual client's communication skills. Furthermore, current approaches focus on helping the hearing-impaired person make optimal use of acoustic cues regardless of the assistive device worn. What has evolved is an extension of previous approaches designed for use with hearing aids to currently available technology such as cochlear implants and vibrotactile assistive devices. Consistent with this evolution and this chapter's point of view, the definition of auditory training is expanded to encompass *all avenues of stimulation—i.e., auditory, electrical, and vibrotactile.*

64

While audiologists continue to discuss the value of formal auditory training (Fleming, 1972), the form it should take (Davis and Hardick, 1981; Sanders, 1982; Schow et al., 1978) and, finally, its lasting effects (Rubinstein and Boothroyd, 1987), most seem to agree that, for the profoundly late-hearing–impaired person newly fit with an assistive device, some form of auditory training should be a part of the aural rehabilitation program. The most recent and convincing data to support this premise can be found in Rubinstein and Boothroyd (1987). They studied 20 adults with mild-to-moderate sensorineural hearing impairment under several training conditions and concluded that:

. . . results of this study support the inclusion of some type of formal auditory training in programs of aural rehabilitation with adults, although they do not support use of a particular training method. The results also demonstrate that gains achieved through training are not lost at least during the period immediately following the end of training (pp. 158-159).

SPEECH PERCEPTION SKILLS ASSESSMENT

A number of tests have been developed to assess the use of the minimal residual auditory abilities in a severely or profoundly impaired individual. These tests were developed to accomplish goals that conventional word recognition tasks do not. They measure the capability of residual hearing beyond an all-or-none (correct/incorrect) response by providing structured situations (closed sets) and simple stimuli such as sentences coordinated to a printed list. The tests vary greatly in task difficulty, the more vigorous requiring fine analysis of auditory cues. The simplest tasks require recognition or discrimination of gross aspects of the signal.

A measure that has gained widespread use is the Minimal Auditory Capabilities (MAC) Battery (Owens, Kessler, and Telleen et al., 1981; Owens et al., 1983). Subtests of the MAC examine the person's ability to discriminate between questions vs. statements, noise vs. voice, and closed sets of spondees. Other subtests include recognition of environmental sounds and locus of "accent" in sentences. The authors devised printed materials coordinated with the tests so that printed instructions and answer sets (for closed sets) are available. This battery permits the examiner to be analytic about the types of abilities the patient can use effectively and provides indication of a possible pattern of dysfunction. Our patients' performance on selected subtests of the MAC Battery appears in Table 3-1.

Fine analysis of speech perception skills, including perception of stress or distinctive features, may be obtained by administration of the Speech Pattern Contrast (SPAC) Test (Boothroyd, 1984; 1987), the Iowa Medial Consonant Test (Tyler, Preece, and Lowder, 1983) or the Diagnostic Rhyme Test (DRT) (Voiers et al., 1961; Olroyd, 1972; Voiers, 1977). The SPAC allows examination of roving stress, pitch and intonation, vowel height and place, initial consonant voicing and con-

TABLE 3-1   Mean performance and quartile ranges on Minimal Auditory Capabilities (MAC) Battery

MAC subtests	N	X̄	SD	Quartile cut-off 25th	Quartile cut-off 75th
Question/statement	13	12.08	5.30	10	17
Vowel	8	32.88	11.85	29	44
Spondee recognition	8	7.38	6.93	0	10
Noise/voice	19	30.21	6.72	26	36
Accent	8	11.38	4.34	6	14
Spondee same/different	25	14.84	5.84	9	18

TABLE 3-2   Mean performance and quartile ranges on Diagnostic Rhyme Test (DRT)*

Feature	N	X̄	SD	Quartile cut-off 25th	Quartile cut-off 75th
Voicing	10	28.90	40.73	0	63
Nasality	10	53.90	38.66	25	88
Sustention	10	22.50	35.66	0	63
Sibilation	10	23.10	34.42	6	31
Graveness	10	7.70	17.98	−6	19
Compactness	10	31.30	21.59	19	44
Total Score	10	27.90	27.01	3	53

*In percent correct, corrected for guessing.

tinuance, final consonant voicing and continuance, consonant place, and phoneme recognition. Such fine aspects of recognition performance may be used to construct drill materials to improve specific components of performance. Such exercises may be particularly relevant to a high-functioning patient.

The DRT provides a distinctive feature analysis for nasality, voicing, sustention, sibilance, graveness, and compactness. The test is constructed as a two-alternative forced choice paradigm. In our program, we produced our own audio and videotape versions of this test (Milner and Flevaris-Phillips, 1985). In Table 3-2, we summarize the findings on the DRT for our patients. These scores are corrected for guessing so that a value of 0% indicates no discrimination beyond random guessing. It is interesting to examine how performance may change for various features following fitting with an assistive device and over time with training. This procedure, too, may be useful to the clinician in selecting phonemic content for drill materials.

Another, more difficult, type of auditory assessment material was developed in England—the Bamford, Kowal, and Bench (BKB) Sentences (Bench and Bamford, 1973). The latter materials are composed of sentences administered in a background of competing noise at adverse signal-to-noise ratios. Ability to perform sentence level tasks in quiet, but with breakdown in function during noise, provides the clinician with a high level starting point for therapeutic trials. Such assessment and training protocols in noise and quiet have also been suggested by Garstecki (1984).

On a more basic level, it is necessary for some adults with late-onset deafness to use simpler paradigms, which were originally described in the literature to evaluate deaf children. For example, the Monosyllable-Trochee-Spondee (MTS) test (Erber and Alencewicz, 1976) provides insight into gross discrimination among a closed set of words of one or two syllables. Failure to perform above chance for recognition of specific stimuli or differentiation among the three stress patterns is an indication of dysfunction that implies training should begin at the earliest level of our hierarchy.

Another measure that provides results indicating level of auditory ability is the Test of Auditory Comprehension (TAC) (Trammell, Farrar, Frances et al., 1980) developed for use with children or young adults. The TAC consists of ten subtests that assess reception of a wide variety of speech and nonspeech signals, including some stereotypic phrases. The TAC stimuli progress in complexity from subtest to subtest. The level at which the patient fails provides guidance to rehabilitative needs.

UTILITY OF VIBROTACTILE DEVICES

While most clinicians are quite familiar with the numerous types and models of hearing aid and cochlear implant devices, many may not be as familiar with *vibrotactile* devices. Consequently a brief discussion of these devices seems in order.

Vibrotactile stimulation devices present the acoustic speech stimulus in a vibratory form to the sense of feeling rather than hearing. Vibrotactile devices typically consist of a powerful body-type amplifier or signal processor with either a single vibrator or array of small vibrators attached by a harness or a velcro strip to the client's wrist, hand, chest or back, providing tactile stimulation of the skin. The acoustic speech stimulus is converted into vibratory patterns directly related to the acoustic wave that strikes the microphone of the device, which in turn provides cues that assist in determining the rate and rhythm of speech or, through multiple channels, pitch information. Contemporary devices include as many as 16 contiguous frequency-band channels. The output of each band is presented to a different place on the skin, allowing for more definitive analysis of the acoustic stimulus.

Because vibrotactile sense has limitations in its ability to differentiate the acoustic spectrum of speech, these devices are used primarily to supplement audition and vision. They are used with profoundly hearing-impaired individuals who cannot benefit from acoustic amplification or a cochlear implant. Should a vibrotactile device be indicated, extensive training in learning to use the device is in order. The therapy methods presented in this book are generic and apply to all stimulation devices and, therefore, have direct application to this type of stimulation training. Some authors, such as Youdelman and Behrman (1986), have developed additional training materials for vibrotactile devices.

TELEPHONE TRAINING

For most of society the use of the telephone is a normal part of everyday communication activity and is taken for granted. Most people can communicate freely with the person on the other end of the telephone line and conduct social and/or business transactions with reasonable success. This is not true for the late-deafened adult. For many of these individuals, the telephone is unavailable to them unless some attempt is made to help them compensate for the fact that their profound hearing impairment renders speech on the telephone nearly or completely unintelligible. This is especially true for the new cochlear implantee or user of another recently acquired listening device. Improved telephone communication skills can be achieved with systematic training in the use of the telephone (Erber, 1985).

Castle (1978) described four general approaches typically used by those hearing-impaired individuals who do try to communicate using the telephone. The approach used is governed to a great degree by the severity of the hearing loss and the person's hearing impairment history. The four approaches can be summarized as follows:

1. The use of a telecommunication device for the deaf, referred to as a TDD system. The TDD system makes use of teleprinter equipment, which is available to both persons involved in the telephone conversation. The entire conversation takes place through typewritten messages carried across telephone lines.
2. The use of a third person, who does all the talking on the telephone on behalf of the hearing-impaired person and acts as an oral interpreter for the hearing-impaired person.
3. The actual use of the telephone by the hearing-impaired person, who speaks directly to the person who is being called.
4. The actual use of the telephone as in No. 3 with prearranged code-response patterns.

There are advantages and disadvantages to each of these approaches. The TDD requires that each person involved in the telephone conversation have access to the electronic device, while the "oral interpreter" approach limits the hearing-impaired person's privacy and renders him/her dependent on someone else to use the telephone. Although these two approaches are superior to complete non-use of the telephone, the interactive characteristics of the third and fourth approaches are preferable and have become the focus of many telephone communication training procedures (Erber, 1985).

The third approach is appropriate for someone whose hearing configuration is such that it lends itself to understanding enough of the spoken message via the telephone so that, with practice, successful communication can take place. This approach can be made applicable to persons with profound hearing loss, but it is more successful with persons who have better hearing. In selected cases, telephone communication has been successfully regained with all three of the assistive devices discussed. Nevertheless, the fourth approach is most applicable to the profoundly hearing-impaired person who is the subject of this book. Erber describes the approach as follows:

A profoundly hearing-impaired person may learn to initiate and then guide the direction and content of the conversation. A conversation may take the following form: the hearing impaired person (usually) asks a series of questions that have yes or no answers, and the hearing person at the other end of the telephone line responds with one of several pre-arranged messages that differ in intensity pattern (e.g., "No"—one syllable; "That's "OK," or "Yes, yes"—two syllables; or "I do not understand your speech; please repeat"—many syllables) (p. 14).

Erber (1985) describes the main components of a telephone instruction program: (1) to establish goals, screen abilities, and evaluate the hearing-impaired person's potential for telephone communication; (2) to practice simulated (parts of) conversations, judge success, and practice component skills, if necessary; and (3) to participate in conversations in practical real-life situations. He outlines numerous possibilities for improving communication by telephone (see the box on p. 70). For further discussion of the topic, the reader is referred to Erber's complete text and most especially to Chapter 8, which focuses on the target population of this book.

RESOURCES FOR ADDITIONAL AUDITORY TRAINING MATERIALS

There have been other teams working parallel to ours who have developed many worthwhile auditory training materials.

WAYS TO IMPROVE SPEECH COMMUNICATION OVER A TELEPHONE FOR HEARING-IMPAIRED PEOPLE

Telephone apparatus

Increase the frequency range of the telephone system
Reduce noise and distortion in the telephone system
Transmit visible speech information over ordinary telephone lines*

Hearing aids

Reduce distortion in hearing aids
Improve hearing aid design and selection procedures
Optimize coupling between the telephone and the hearing aid

Information

Learn more about one's own hearing abilities and limitations
Anticipate predictable confusion
Learn about typical conversational sequences
Learn how to simplify the conversational format
Learn techniques for guiding conversations

Strategies

Select or create a quiet environment
Use listening devices appropriately
Plan messages
Choose message form (i.e., vocabulary and syntax) and content (i.e., topic) for high
   potential intelligibility
Apply or request strategies for initial utterance (simple, redundant)
Apply or request strategies for clarification of utterance (louder, rephrase)
Apply message confirmation techniques
Write parts of message when received as a memory aid (have pencil and paper
   handy)
Select talker for optimal voice and articulation qualities, when possible
Persistently guide talker's speech and language output
Inform the public how they can help a hearing-impaired person during a telephone
   conversation

---

*As technology becomes available, video telephone should be made available to facilitate speech-reading.
From Erber NP: *Telephone communication and hearing impairment,* San Diego, 1985, College-Hill Press, p. 16.

A group at the National Acoustics Laboratory (NAL) has developed the following training packages: A Communication Training Program for Profoundly Deafened Adults, COMMTRAM (Plant, 1984); Modified Connected Discourse Tracking Exercise for Hearing-Impaired Adults, COMMTRAC (Plant, 1989); and Synthetic Training Exercises for Hearing-Impaired Adults, SYNTREX (Plant, 1991). The NAL materials give ample, interesting story and conversational style exercises at an adult level.

Most inventive clinicians recognize that maintaining interest in the therapy situation can be a difficult challenge. As indicated in our therapy plans, the use of commercially manufactured games without speechreading cues (e.g., *Trivial Pursuit, Clue, Pictionary, Bingo,* card games) can provide a nonthreatening method for practice. Such games have a high demand for accurate information transmission and reception, as well as promoting guessing and synthesis of clues and observations.

We have also provided a narrative, "Ideas for Home Therapy" (Appendix A). Many of our patients have been interested in practicing their new auditory skills at home. Our handout encourages the patient to continue at home with a partner using the speechtracking techniques learned in the clinic. For auditory training purposes, such shadowing can be done in a listening-only mode (i.e., without lipreading).

We have also encouraged patients to try listening to audiotaped books, such as those recorded for the blind. However, sometimes, these materials may be recorded at a rate that is unsuitable for the hearing impaired, and the patient should be warned about this potential problem. Such recordings offer the option of choosing materials of individual interest and frequently have the advantage of coordinated text available. There are also recordings of environmental sounds, which may be of interest to some patients. If the books for the visually impaired are too difficult or too rapid for a given patient, it is possible to use recordings for children, in which the rate is generally slower and the linguistic level less complex.

Consistent with this text's theme, all telephone training should begin with a systematic diagnostic procedure. Appendix B contains one such procedure, the "Component Scale for Assessing Use of Telecommunication Devices," developed specifically for this project (Spitzer, unpublished). The scale assesses the patient's ability to use the telephone effectively in conjunction with the assistive device. For example, it determines whether the patient is accurate and comfortable in juxtaposing the telephone and the assistive device and manipulating its switches, or whether the various signals of the telephone (ringing, busy signal, answering) can be detected with consistency. The scale provides both open- and closed-set material.

THERAPY PLANS: GOALS, OBJECTIVES, AND SUCCESS CRITERIA

The lesson plans outlined in this chapter are generic in design and are intended to be adaptable to acoustic, electrical, or vibrotactile stimulation. They address the perception of six basic stimuli (i.e., voice, environmental sounds, number of syllables, acoustic prosody, vowel position, and consonant position). The activities are centered around the easier listening task of detection (the presence or absence of a signal) and progress to the more difficult tasks of discrimination (are two signals the same or different?) and identification (also known as recognition). The use of visual cues is suggested whenever possible so that the stimuli are presented as naturally as possible. The protocol includes the use of both the "open-set" (unlimited number of choices) and the "closed-set" (limited number of choices) approaches. It is suggested, however, that the "closed-set" approach be employed as often as is needed to ensure early and sustained success with the speech perception activities.

The following goals and objectives are meant to provide the aural rehabilitationist with a prescriptive approach to the rehabilitation of persons with a severe or profound hearing impairment. The activities are categorized by level of difficulty, starting with the level of least difficulty.

The protocol is based on a series of goals, objectives, procedures, and criterion measures. Goals are based on certain aspects of various diagnostic tests used to assess the auditory functioning and rehabilitative needs of the individual. These auditory tests include the MAC Battery, the Iowa Test Battery, the MTS test, and the DRT described earlier in this chapter.

A. GOAL: To *perceive* voice.

  1. Objective: To *detect* voice under quiet conditions with assistive device set to most comfortable listening level.

   Procedure: A stimulus will consist of either a male voice or female voice recorded under quiet conditions. Introduce stimulus or silent interval using an irregular schedule. The examiner will cue the patient when a listening trial is about to begin. A response should indicate the presence or absence of voice.

   Criterion: Clinician monitoring—90% success rate.

   Materials: Tape recordings of female and male voices with and without background noise. Use of commercially available recorded stimulus acceptable. (Materials same for Objectives 2 to 5, Goal A.)

  2. Objective: To *discriminate* voice under quiet conditions with assistive device set to most comfortable listening level.

Procedure: Stimuli will consist of a series of voices. Introduce two stimuli. A stimulus pair will consist of either male voices, female voices, or a male/female combination. A response will indicate the two stimuli as the same or different.

Criterion: Clinician monitoring—90% success rate.

3. **Objective**: To *identify* gender of voice under quiet conditions with assistive device set to most comfortable listening level.

    Procedure: Introduce one stimulus. The stimulus will consist of a male or female voice. Several different speakers are recommended. Response should indicate voice is perceived as male or female.

    Criterion: Clinician monitoring—90% success rate.

4. **Objective**: To *identify* speaker under quiet conditions with assistive device set to most comfortable listening level.

    Procedure: Tape recordings of the voices of significant others and familiar individuals will be presented. A response will indicate the identity of the person speaking.

    Criterion: Clinician monitoring—90% success rate.

5. **Objective**: To *achieve* the previous objectives in the presence of varying degrees of background noise (e.g., multi-talker babble, cafeteria noise, or white noise). If responses remain consistently high, level of background noise may be increased until patient is challenged.

    Procedure: As outlined previously.

    Criterion: As outlined previously.

B. **GOAL**: To *perceive* environmental sounds using auditory input only.

1. **Objective**: To *detect* environmental sounds under quiet conditions with assistive device set to most comfortable listening level.

    Procedure: Stimulus will consist of various environmental sounds recorded under quiet conditions. Introduce stimulus or silent interval using an irregular schedule. Examiner cues the patient when a listening trial is about to begin. Response should indicate the presence or absence of a sound.

    Criterion: Clinical monitoring—90% success rate.

    Materials: Tape recordings of various types of environmental sounds. (Materials same for Objectives 2 to 4, Goal B.)

2. **Objective**: To *discriminate* environmental sounds under quiet conditions with assistive device set to most comfortable listening level.

    Procedure: Introduce two stimuli. A stimulus pair should consist of a combination of the various types of environmental sounds on tape. Response should indicate the two stimuli as the same or different.

    Criterion: Clinician monitoring—90% success rate.

3. **Objective:** To *identify* environmental sounds under quiet conditions with assistive device set to most comfortable listening level.

    Procedure: Introduce one stimulus. The stimulus should consist of the various types of environmental sounds available on tape. Response should indicate the type of sound perceived using a closed-set format. Once this has been satisfactorily achieved, an open-set format should be employed.

    Criterion: Clinician monitoring—90% success rate.

4. **Objective:** To *achieve* the previous objectives in the presence of varying degrees of background noise (e.g., multi-talker babble, cafeteria noise, or white noise). If responses remain consistently high, level of background noise may be increased until patient is challenged.

    Procedure: As outlined previously.

    Criterion: As outlined previously.

C. **GOAL:** To *perceive* words as varying in the number of syllables (one, two, or three).

1. **Objective:** To *define* the differences between monosyllables, spondees and trochees, and three-syllable words.

    Procedure: Didactic presentation of the different types of words (i.e., one vs. two vs. three-syllable words). Contrast spondee and trochee words. Highlight the importance of understanding such differences as they relate to improved speech reception. Open discussion; ongoing.

    Criterion: Patient demonstrates understanding by conversation with the clinician.

    Materials: Definitions and illustrations of what constitute monosyllable, spondee, trochee, and three-syllable words; also examples following, presented using live voice or tape recordings (see also pp. 69 and 71 for additional resources for similar materials).

2. **Objective:** To *detect* silence and monosyllable, spondee, trochee, and three-syllable words using live voice or tape recorded material under quiet conditions with assistive device set to most comfortable listening level.

    Procedure: Present monosyllable, spondee, trochee, and three-syllable words in random order. Response will indicate signal as present or absent. If the criterion is not achieved using acoustic cues only, use visual cues.

    Criterion: Clinician monitoring—90% success rate.

    Materials:

Monosyllable	Spondee	Trochee	Three syllable
plan	baseball	climber	nutrition
block	cloudburst	neon	nursery
horse	whitewash	after	equator

Monosyllable	Spondee	Trochee	Three syllable
boat	horseshoe	tempest	disputed
cow	wishbone	compare	temperature
eel	railroad	vampire	opposite
sun	pigtail	blossom	gazebo
play	starship	wagon	dignity
gaze	playground	pervert	allocate
tag	treehouse	nostril	cathedral
ant	mushroom	petal	volleyball
dog	hardware	lantern	nominee
lamp	headlight	carton	atrophy
white	iceberg	carpet	integrate
air	cowboy	downsize	trespassing
grass	earmark	sickness	lawnmower
fish	whitewash	thankful	glossary
please	hotdog	frigid	equation
no	doorknob	liquid	porcupine
hair	armchair	chaos	masterful
rope	sidewalk	housework	synonym
tree	cupcake	coldcuts	vestibule
I	limestone	westward	abdicate
show	downtown	turnstile	constitute
pain	outside	standing	spectator
land	lighthouse	equal	dehydrate
bug	ice cream	doggie	contemplate
fur	hitchhike	peaceful	disfigure
soft	witchcraft	hobby	blasphemy
bride	iceberg	middle	consider
dust	hightail	fender	disorder
duck	earthworm	nearly	powerless
hole	ski trail	reptile	unequal
tail	landscape	cheetah	miserly
sit	checkroom	fearless	quarterly
coin	starlight	happy	afterward
ride	rundown	hunger	bicycle
find	bedspread	baby	cottontail
sack	bathmat	beauty	betrayal
bag	hillside	garbage	photograph

3. **Objective:** To *discriminate* monosyllable, spondee, trochee, and three-syllable words under quiet conditions with assistive device set to most comfortable listening level.

Procedure: Introduce randomized word pairs consisting of one- two- or three-syllable words. Response will indicate words as same or different based on number of syllables only. If the criterion is not readily achieved using acoustic cues only, use visual cues.

Criterion: Clinician monitoring—90% success rate.

Materials:

Monosyllable	Spondee	Trochee	Three syllable
build	field trip	seesaw	sensible
gold	stoneware	pastry	practical
nest	stove pipe	forest	runaway
sad	sales clerk	landmark	luxury
gift	skin graft	rumpus	handicraft
truck	spacecraft	snowdrift	sadistic
hand	oneway	onion	satisfy
witch	shortcake	warthog	opium
crack	old world	often	temptation
Greek	lone shark	complex	temperance
ooze	guesswork	remark	lunatic
thumb	hayfork	loveless	lopsided
sell	grapefruit	cobra	hospital
boy	daybreak	erect	dislocate
dart	shorthand	modern	sunglasses
leaf	landmark	tangle	detector
head	postmark	dismiss	snowmobile
bird	ice tea	placemat	pumpkin pie
bell	dartboard	crumble	velvety
dad	cut throat	suspense	daffodil

4. **Objective:** To *identify* monosyllable, spondee, trochee, and three-syllable words under quiet conditions with assistive device set to most comfortable listening level.

   Procedure: Introduce a word. Response will indicate number of syllables in the word. Once this objective has satisfactorily been achieved, response should indicate the word spoken, using first a closed-set format progressing to an open-set format. If the criterion is not readily achieved using acoustic cues only, use visual cues.

   Criterion: Clinician monitoring—90% success rate.

   Materials: Use word lists from Objectives 2 and 3.

5. **Objective:** To *achieve* the previous objectives in the presence of low ambient noise, gradually decreasing non-acoustic cues until total reliance is on auditory input only.

   Procedure: As outlined previously.

   Criterion: As outlined previously.

   Materials: As outlined previously.

D. GOAL: To *perceive* spondee and trochee words.

1. **Objective:** To *discriminate* spondee and trochee words under quiet conditions with assistive device set to most comfortable listening level.

   Procedure: Introduce words from the lists given in the section on materials. Patient is to indicate if the word presented is a spondee or trochee.

Criterion: Clinician monitoring—90% success rate.
Materials:

Spondee	Trochee
ground crew	beetle
network	impale
knowhow	upset
nosebleed	crowded
kneejerk	detour
airplane	taco
mushroom	sentence
knicknack	clover
knockdown	cradle
nightgown	sister
nightmare	entrance
star drive	apple
raincoat	weekend
packhorse	jockey
buckboard	pickup
starlight	ransom
stagecoach	playful
busboy	monarch
framework	worthless
birthmark	tripod
earwax	tremble
dancewear	custom

2. **Objective:** To *identify* spondee and trochee words with assistive device set to most comfortable listening level.
   Procedure: Introduce spondee and trochee words. Response will indicate which stress pattern (spondee or trochee) has been presented. Use an open-set format unless the patient encounters difficulty. If patient cannot reach the criterion readily, use closed set and/or supplement with visual cues.
   Criterion: Clinician monitoring—90% success rate.
   Materials: Use spondee and trochee lists from Objectives 2 and 3, Goal C and Objective 1, Goal D.
3. **Objective:** To *recognize* spondee and trochee words with assistive device set to most comfortable listening level.
   Procedure: As outlined previously.
   Criterion: As outlined previously.
   Materials: As outlined previously.
4. **Objective:** To *achieve* the previous objectives in the presence of low ambient noise, gradually decreasing non-acoustic cues until total reliance is on auditory input only.
   Procedure: As outlined previously.

Criterion: As outlined previously.

Materials: As outlined previously.

E. GOAL: To *perceive* the acoustic cues associated with prosody.

1. Objective: To *understand* the role that acoustic cues play in everyday communication, (i.e., define frequency [pitch], intensity [loudness], and duration [length] as they relate to speech perception).

Procedure: Discuss how frequency, intensity, and duration interact to relay a communicative intent. Include aspects of the attributes that interact on both the sentence and word level. Open discussion; ongoing.

Criterion: Patient demonstrates understanding by conversation with the clinician.

Materials: Definitions of prosody to include discussion of frequency, intensity, duration, stress, and accent; sentences of varying length (see Chapter 5); and word pairs (see Objective 1, Goal D). Materials should be kept pertinent to patient's needs as well as preferences. (Materials the same for Objectives 2 to 10, Goal E.)

2. Objective: To *detect* stress of words within the context of a sentence under quiet conditions with assistive device set to most comfortable listening level.

Procedure: Present in random order a four-word sentence with or without stress. When using stress, randomly choose the one word to be stressed. Response must indicate the presence or absence of stress. For patients fitted with a cochlear implant, vibrotactile device, or powerful body aid, it is necessary to provide them with a copy of the sentences being presented. If criterion is not readily met, use visual cues.

Criterion: Clinician monitoring—90% success rate.

3. Objective: To *discriminate* differences in stress at the sentence level under quiet conditions with assistive device set to most comfortable listening level.

Procedure: Present the same sentence twice, with either the same or contrastive stress pattern. Response must indicate the same or different based on the stress pattern of the sentence. For patients fitted with a cochlear implant, vibrotactile device, or powerful body aid, it is necessary to provide them with a copy of the sentences to be recited. Use of visual cues is permissible to obtain correct responses.

Criterion: Clinician monitoring—90% success rate.

4. Objective: To *identify* differences in stress at the sentence level under quiet conditions with assistive device set to most comfortable listening level.

Procedure: Present a sentence. Stress one word in the sentence. Response should indicate which word was stressed. For patients fitted with a cochlear

implant, vibrotactile device, or powerful body aid, it is necessary to provide them with a copy of the sentences to be recited. Use of visual cues is
permissible to obtain correct responses.

Criterion: Clinician monitoring—90% success rate.

5. **Objective:** To *achieve* the previous objectives in the presence of low ambient noise, gradually decreasing non-acoustic cues until total reliance is
on auditory input only.

   Procedure: As outlined previously.

   Criterion: As outlined previously.

6. **Objective:** To *define* sentences, such as statements, questions, exclamations and imperatives, based on acoustic differences in frequency, intensity, and duration.

   Procedure: Discuss acoustic differences among sentences and how the
acoustic information is used to relay communicative intent. Discuss all
types of sentences but focus on two types—statements and questions. Open
discussion; ongoing.

   Criterion: Patient demonstrates understanding by conversation with the
clinician.

7. **Objective:** To *detect* the acoustic patterns associated with statements and
questions under quiet conditions with assistive device set to most comfortable listening level.

   Procedure: Focus on one sentence type at a time. Indicate sentence type
under discussion. Present a series of four-word stimuli. Response will indicate when a target sentence-type (question or statement) has been heard.
Use of visual cues is permissible to obtain correct responses.

   Criterion: Clinician monitoring—90% success rate.

8. **Objective:** To *discriminate* the acoustic patterns associated with statements
and questions under quiet conditions with assistive device set to most comfortable listening level.

   Procedure: Introduce two four-word sentences (see pp. 69 and 71 for resources for additional auditory training materials). Response will indicate
the sentences as same or different based on the acoustic patterns. Use of
visual cues is permissible to obtain correct responses.

   Criterion: Clinician monitoring—90% success rate.

9. **Objective:** To *identify* the acoustic attributes associated with statements,
questions, exclamations, and imperatives under quiet conditions with assistive device set to most comfortable listening level.

   Procedure: Introduce a sentence. Response should indicate the type of sentence spoken. If criterion is not readily met, use of visual cues is permissible to obtain correct responses.

   Criterion: Clinician monitoring—90% success rate.

10. **Objective:** To *achieve* the previous objectives in the presence of low am-

bient noise, gradually decreasing the non-acoustic cues until total reliance is on auditory input only.

Procedure: As outlined previously.

Criterion: As outlined previously.

F. GOAL: To *perceive* three vowels at the extremes of the vowel triangle (i.e., /i,u,a/).

1. Objective: To *review* vowels and their acoustic attributes.

Procedure: Discuss the frequency and intensity composition of vowels and the roles they play in speech reception. Open discussion; ongoing.

Criterion: Patient demonstrates understanding by conversation with the clinician.

Materials: Lists of words representing the three vowel types. (Materials same for Objectives 2, 4, and 5, Goal F.)

/i/

beak	keep	beet	seed
greet	deal	seen	feet
keen	bean	seat	lead
fleet	lean	seal	green
beam	treat	meat	seam
cheat	deed	mean	weed

/u/

noon	boost	food	broom
tune	maroon	loon	flew
roost	stew	gloom	boot
glue	goose	balloon	hoop
boom	racoon	soup	poodle
moon	loose	root	blue

/a/

pot	crock	toddler	flop
lock	top	pop	sock
got	not	drop	rock
hot	mop	bond	fox
rot	coddle	box	doctor
lottery	bottle	clock	hop

2. Objective: To *detect* the three different vowels in real one-syllable words under quiet conditions with the assistive device set to most comfortable listening level.

Procedure: Indicate vowel under discussion. Response must indicate the presence or absence of the particular vowel. Procedure is repeated for each vowel. If criterion is not readily achieved, use visual cues.

Criterion: Clinician monitoring—90% success rate.

3. **Objective:** To *discriminate* the three vowels under quiet conditions with assistive device set to most comfortable listening level.

   Procedure: Present word pairs. Response must indicate whether the vowel occurring is the same or different. If criterion is not met, use of visual cues is permissible to obtain correct responses.

   Criterion: Clinician monitoring—90% success rate.

   Materials: Word lists in Objective 1 or those in *Nucleus 22 Channel Cochlear Implant System Rehabilitation Manual* (Mecklenburg et al., 1987).

4. **Objective:** To *identify* the three vowels under quiet conditions with assistive device set to most comfortable listening level.

   Procedure: Present a word with a previously identified vowel (open set). Response must indicate which vowel occurred. Once this objective has been satisfactorily achieved, response should indicate not only the vowel but also the word. If the criterion is not readily met, use of visual cues is permissible to obtain correct responses.

   Criterion: Clinician monitoring—90% success rate.

5. **Objective:** To *achieve* the previous objectives in the presence of low ambient noise, gradually decreasing the non-acoustic cues until total reliance is on auditory input only.

   Procedure: As outlined previously.

   Criterion: As outlined previously.

G. **GOAL:** To *perceive* consonants in varying positions.

1. **Objective:** To *review* consonants and their acoustic attributes.

   Procedure: Discuss the frequency and intensity composition of consonants and the role they play in speech reception. Open discussion; ongoing.

   Criterion: Patient demonstrates understanding by conversation with the clinician.

   Materials: Lists of words in isolation and in pairs, using a text such as *40,000 Selected Words* (Blockcolsky et al., 1987). (Materials same for Objectives 2 to 6, Goal G.)

2. **Objective:** To *detect* consonants in final, initial, and medial position under quiet conditions with assistive device set to most comfortable listening level.

   Procedure: Indicate consonant and position under discussion. Begin trials with most visible consonants and progress toward less visible consonants. Present words with consonant in appropriate position. Response must indicate the presence or absence of the consonant in the position being discussed. Use of gestures and facial expressions is permissible to obtain correct responses.

Criterion: Clinician monitoring—90% success rate.

3. **Objective:** To *discriminate* consonants in final, initial, and medial position under quiet conditions with assistive device set to most comfortable listening level.

   Procedure: Indicate consonant position under discussion. Present a word pair containing the same consonant in the same or different position. Response must indicate whether the consonant occurred in the same or different position. Use of gestures and facial expressions is permissible to obtain correct responses.

   Criterion: Clinician monitoring—90% success rate.

4. **Objective:** To *identify* consonants in final, initial, and medial position under quiet conditions with assistive device set to most comfortable listening level. It is important to emphasize the consonants based on their categorization, namely voicing, nasality, fricatives, glides, semiglides, and stop plosives. This class system may be more readily intelligible to the patient than that of Voiers et al. (1977) (see p. 66).

   Procedure: Present a word. Instruct individual to indicate the consonant presented and the position in which it occurs. Once this objective has been satisfactorily achieved, response should indicate not only the consonant and position, but also the word presented. A closed-set format is suggested initially with progression to an open-set format. Use of gestures and facial expressions is permissible to obtain correct responses.

   Criterion: Clinician monitoring—90% success rate.

5. **Objective:** To *achieve* the previous objectives, gradually decreasing non-acoustic cues until total reliance is on auditory input only.

   Procedure: As outlined previously.

   Criterion: As outlined previously.

6. **Objective:** To *achieve* the previous objectives in the presence of low ambient noise, gradually decreasing non-acoustic cues until total reliance is on auditory input only.

   Procedure: As outlined previously.

   Criterion: As outlined previously.

H. GOAL: To *develop* maximal use of assistive device in conjunction with the telephone.

1. **Objective:** To *train* how to interface assistive device with the telephone.

   Procedure: Demonstration and practice in coupling and uncoupling the assistive device to the telephone. Teaching the appropriate use of assistive device's switches and cables.

   Criterion: Patient demonstrates understanding by conversation with the clinician.

Materials: Telephone and assistive device assessed by factor 1, *Component Scale* (Appendix B).

2. **Objective:** *Review* of the pragmatics of telephone conversations.
   Procedure: Training and practice in detection and recognition of telephone signals (i.e., dial tone, ringing, busy signal, telephone being answered.) To review and practice conversational turn-taking and detection of conversational partner's voice.
   Criterion: 90% success rate on factor 2, *Component Scale* (Appendix B).
   Materials: Telephone signals and normal conversations.

3. **Objective:** To *develop* ability to use telephone codes.
   Procedure: Describe code used to the patient. Specifically, when the telephone receiver is picked up and the call is answered, the patient should recognize that the ring has ceased and the recipient has said "Hello." The patient will then say, "Hello, I am (Name) and am hearing impaired. I can understand you on the telephone if we follow some basic rules. I will ask you questions in order to obtain the information I need, and you will answer in the following way: To say 'no,' simply say 'no' one time. To say 'yes,' always say 'yes, yes.' If you do not follow my question, say, 'I don't understand,' and I will ask the question again or in a different way. Are we ready to begin?" The clinician and the patient then practice the procedure on the telephone in the office.
   Criterion: 90% success rate on factor 3, *Component Scale* (Appendix B).
   Materials: Two telephones in an office and closed-set message forms A and B, *Phone Conversation with a Friend: Sending a Message* (Appendix B).

4. **Objective:** To *develop* ability to obtain open-set information over the telephone.
   Procedure: Practice conversation on the telephone with (a) topic known and (b) topic unknown.
   Criterion: 90% success rate on factor 4, *Component Scale* (Appendix B).
   Materials: Two telephones in an office and open-set message forms A and B, *Phone Conversation with a Friend: Receiving a Message* (Appendix B).

5. **Objective:** To *develop* confidence in use of the telephone.
   Procedure: Discussion of strategies and ways to improve ease and frequency of telephone conversations.
   Criterion: 90% success rate on factor 5, *Component Scale* (Appendix B).
   Materials: Two telephones in an office and *Component Scale* (Appendix B) and *Feelings about Telecommunication* (Appendix C).

REFERENCES

Anderson SW, editor: *Cochlear prostheses: an international symposium,* New York, 1983, New York Academy of Sciences.

Bench J, Bamford J: *Speech-hearing tests and the spoken language of hearing-impaired children,* London, 1973, Academic Press.

Blockcolsky VD, Frazer JM, Frazer DH: *40,000 Selected Words,* Tuscon, Ariz, 1979, Communication Skill Builders.

Boothroyd A: Auditory perception of speech contrasts by subjects with sensorineural hearing loss, *J Speech Hear Res* 27:338-352, 1984.

Boothroyd A: Perception of speech contrasts via cochlear implants and limited hearing, *Ann Otol Rhinol Laryngol* 96(suppl 128):58-62, 1987.

Davis JM, Hardick, EJ: *Rehabilitive audiology for children and adults,* New York, 1981, John Wiley & Sons.

Erber NP: Ways to improve speech communication over a telephone for hearing-impaired people. In Erber NP: *Telephone communication and hearing impairment,* San Diego, 1985, College-Hill Press.

Erber NP, Alencewicz CA: Audiologic evaluation of deaf children, *J Speech Hear Dis* 41:256-267, 1976.

Flemming M: A total approach to communication therapy, *J Acad Rehab Audio* 5:28-31, 1972.

Garstecki DC: Rehabilitation of hearing-impaired adults. In Jerger J, editor: *Hearing disorders in adults,* San Diego, 1984, College Hill Press, pp 175-200.

Jeffers J, Barely M: *Speechreading and lipreading,* Springfield, Ill, 1971, Charles C Thomas.

Mecklenburg DJ, Dowell RC, Jenison VW: *Nucleus 22 Channel Cochlear Implant System Rehabilitation Manual,* Denver, 1987, Cochlear Corporation.

Milner P, Flevaris-Phillips C: Speech reception in deaf adult using vibrotactile aids or cochlear implants, *J Acoust Soc Am* 78:517, 1985.

Micolosi L, Harryman E, Kresheck J: *Terminology of communication disorder,* Baltimore, 1978, Williams & Wilkins.

& Wilkins.

Olroyd MH: *Employment of the Diagnostic Rhyme Test (DRT) with normal-hearing and sensorineural hearing-impaired listeners,* doctoral dissertation, 1972, Louisiana State University Microfilms (73-2974).

Owens E, Kessler DK, Raggio M: Results of some patients with cochlear implants on The Minimal Auditory Capabilities Battery. Parkins CW, Anderson SW: *Cochlear Prostheses: An International Symposium,* New York Academy of Sciences, New York, 1983.

Owens E, Kessler DK et al: The Minimal Auditory Capabilities (MAC) Battery, *Hear Aid J* 34:9, 1981.

Plant G: *An auditory training program for the hearing impaired adult,* Sydney, 1981, National Acoustics Laboratory.

Plant G: *COMMTRAM: A Communication Training Program for Profoundly Deafened Adults,* Sydney, 1984, National Acoustics Laboratory.

Plant G: *COMMTRAC: Modified Connected Discourse Tracking for Hearing Impaired Adults,* Sydney, 1989, National Acoustics Laboratory.

Plant G: *SYNTREX: Synthetic Training Exercises for Hearing Impaired Adults,* Sydney, 1991, National Acoustics Laboratory.

Rubenstein A, Boothroyd A: Effect of two approaches to auditory training on speech recognition by hearing-impaired adults, *J Speech Hear Res* 30:153-160, 1987.

Sanders DA: *Aural rehabilitation: a management model,* Englewood Cliffs, NJ, 1982, Prentice-Hall.

Schow RL, Christensen JL, Hutchinson JM et al: *Communication disorders of the aged: a guide for health professionals,* Baltimore, 1978, University Park Press.

Tramell JC, Farrar C, Francis J et al: *Test of auditory comprehension,* California, 1980, Forewords.

Tyler RS, Preece JP, Lowder MW: *The Iowa Cochlear Implant Test,* Iowa City, 1983. University of Iowa Department of Otolaryngology—Head and Neck Surgery.

Voiers WD: Diagnostic evaluation of speech intelligibility. In Hawley ME, editor: *Benchmark papers in acoustics,* vol 11, chapter 34, Stroudsburg, Penn, 1977, Dowden, Hutchinson and Ross.

Voiers WD, Cohen M, Mickunas J: Evaluation of speech processing devices. I. Intelligibility, quality, speaker recognizability, *Final report, contract AF19 (628)4195,* OAS, 1961.

Youdelman K, Behrman AM: *Tactaid manual,* Jackson Heights, NY, 1986, The Lexington Center.

Ideas for Home Therapy

Many of our cochlear implant patients come from so far away that it is not possible to come to our hospital weekly for therapy. It is believed by some cochlear implant specialists that the implantee learns a great deal on his/her own through experience and conversation. Many people, however, do like to practice so we have some suggestions for how you can work on getting the most from your experiences.

Remember that you are learning to listen all over again. Have patience. This is not an overnight change but a gradual learning experience that you will enjoy.

SPEECHTRACKING

Speechtracking is a way of practicing listening. With a partner, you practice using reading materials, such as chapters from an enjoyable book or articles from newspapers or magazines.

There are three parts to this activity. It is done under three conditions:

- Without implant (lipreading only)
- With lipreading and implant together
- With implant only (this is the hardest condition, but you should still try to work at it)

Your partner faces you and reads to you. He/she stops after a phrase and gives you time to repeat what has been said *word for word*. It is very important that you work for 100% accuracy.

If you don't get a word, your partner tells you and gives you clues to help you figure out the correct word. No gestures should be used. It is reasonable to try to give word meanings by illustration with opposites, such as "sounds like . . ." or "means the same as . . ." methods.

You should try this exercise every day if possible. A minimum of 3 to 4 times per week is necessary for consistent practice. It is often best to stick to only one or two partners, especially in the beginning.

LISTENING TO SPOKEN MATERIALS

If you want to try something a little different, go to the library and get out books with accompanying tapes or records. These are especially good when they are tapes developed for the blind and when they are faithful to the text of the original materials, especially novels.

LEARNING SOUNDS IN THE ENVIRONMENT

Sound effects records or tapes are also fun. Get a tape that has a written key, so that you and your partner are sure of what you are listening to.

KEEPING A LOG

It is fun to keep a record of the sounds you hear or the words that you understand. This record should be something like a diary so that you can see how you are adding new sounds as you progress.

APPENDIX B

COMPONENT SCALE FOR ASSESSING USE OF TELECOMMUNICATION DEVICES

The following scale is to be used to assess a patient's ability to convey and obtain information over the telephone.

Factor 1: Knowledge of how to interface the device with the telephone.

Criteria:	NA	WGD				WGE*
• Places the device in correct juxtaposition to phone	0	1	2	3	4	5
• Uses appropriate switches correctly (speed dimension is assessed)	0	1	2	3	4	5

Factor 2: Knowledge of how to begin communication process.

Criteria:

	NA	WGD				WGE
• Can detect (auditorially) various phone signals:						
• Phone ringing	0	1	2	3	4	5
• Busy signal	0	1	2	3	4	5
• Phone answered and begins conversation successfully	0	1	2	3	4	5
OR						
• Cannot detect the above dimensions but can circumnavigate difficulties	0	1	2	3	4	5
OR						
• Successfully uses TDD operator to perform these discriminations and initiates communication successfully	0	1	2	3	4	5

*Factors 1-4: *NA*, not applicable: *WGD*, with great difficulty; *WGE*, with great ease.

Factor 3: Ability to obtain information over the phone: closed-set message.

Factor 3 is assessed by giving the patient a set of questions to which he/she must supply answers, based on calling another extension within the hospital and asking questions of a staff member (see Section I, Form A, pp. 90-91, for stimuli).

In working with a patient with some sophistication, timing responses will give an indication of how *efficiently* information is obtained. Tracking this factor in repeated measurements over time will provide insight regarding increasing facility in telecommunication use.

Criteria:	NA	WGD				WGE
• Uses residual hearing to obtain critical information	0	1	2	3	4	5
• Uses strategy(ies) to obtain information (i.e., to clarify what cannot be heard clearly)	0	1	2	3	4	5
OR						
• Uses a code successfully	0	1	2	3	4	5
OR						
• Uses the TDD efficiently, using abbreviations when appropriate, and asks for information to clarify necessary points (speed dimension is assessed)	0	1	2	3	4	5

Factor 4: Ability to obtain information over the phone: open-set message.

Factor 4 is assessed by having the patient receive a message called in by a staff member (see Section II, Form A, pp. 94-95, for stimuli).

In working with a patient with some sophistication, timing responses will give an indication of how *efficiently* information is obtained. Tracking this factor in repeated measurements over time will provide insight regarding increasing facility in telecommunication use.

Criteria:	NA	WGD				WGE
• Uses residual hearing to obtain critical information	0	1	2	3	4	5
• Uses strategy(ies) to obtain information (i.e., to clarify what cannot be heard clearly)	0	1	2	3	4	5
OR						
• Uses a code successfully	0	1	2	3	4	5
OR						
• Uses the TDD efficiently, using abbreviations when appropriate, and asks for information to clarify necessary points (speed dimension is assessed)	0	1	2	3	4	5

Factor 5: Confidence in telephone use (actual patient response sheet is given in Appendix C).

The patient rates his/her responses to the following statements:

	NA	DS				AS*
• I know that I can use the telephone to obtain the help I would need in an emergency.	0	1	2	3	4	5
• I have great confidence that the information I obtain over the telephone is accurate.	0	1	2	3	4	5
• I enjoy using the telephone to keep in contact with friends and family.	0	1	2	3	4	5
• The telephone is a necessary device in my life.	0	1	2	3	4	5
OR						
• I know that I can use the TDD to obtain the help I would need in an emergency.	0	1	2	3	4	5
• I have great confidence that the information I obtain over the TDD is accurate.	0	1	2	3	4	5
• I enjoy using the TDD to keep in contact with friends and family.	0	1	2	3	4	5
• The TDD is a necessary device in my life.	0	1	2	3	4	5

*Factor 5: *NA*, not applicable; *DS*, disagree strongly; *AS*, agree strongly.

I. PHONE CONVERSATION WITH A FRIEND: SENDING A MESSAGE

Closed-Set Message: Form A

Directions:

Imagine the following situation. You saw a friend last night, and you both agreed to meet sometime soon to go out together. You mentioned a number of possible activities in which you might participate, including bowling, skating, going to the movies, or going to the park for a picnic.

Today you realized that you had not made a definite plan, so you decide to call to firm up what you are doing.

You must obtain answers to the following questions.

1. What activity are you and your friend going to do? _____

2. What day of the week will you go out? _____

3. What time will you go? _____

4. Who else will go with you? _____

5. Where should you meet? _____

6. What do you have to bring with you? _____, _____, ,

7. How (transportation) will you go? _____

8. How much will this activity cost? _____

9. Are you planning on eating out? _____

10. What time will you get home? _____

Response Key for Closed-Set Message: Form A

To be used by phone conversant:

1. Skating

2. Thursday

3. 7:00 PM

4. Your cousin Gene

5. At cousin Gene's house

6. Skates, warm clothes, and tissues

7. By car

8. Two dollars

9. Go out for pizza afterward

10. About 10:00 PM

Accuracy (% correct) score _____ %

Speed score _____ minutes

Closed-Set Message: Form B
Directions:

Imagine the following situation. You are staying at a friend's house for 2 weeks. You would like to contribute to the running of the household while you are visiting. Last night, you noticed that the stock of some food items was low or missing in the kitchen.

Today you realized that you needed to check with your friend about some of the things you would like to buy.

First you must tell your friend about your plan to go shopping. Then obtain answers to the following questions.

1. Does your friend think it's OK for you to do some shopping? _____

2. Where should you go shopping? _____

3. What food items are urgently needed (3 items)? _____,
   _____, _____

4. Are there any special brands for these? _____

5. Are there other, less urgent, things you should buy? _____

6. You would like to make dinner, but what kind of meat does your friend like?
   _____

7. What side dish would he/she like? _____

8. What kind of cake would he/she like for dessert? _____

9. What time should dinner be ready? _____

Response Key for Closed-Set Message: Form B

To be used by phone conversant:

1. Yes, it would be very nice of you to shop.

2. Wadbaum's supermarket

3. Eggs, coffee, milk

4. Yes, coffee should be Chock-Full-O'-Nuts

5. Tunafish and mayonnaise

6. Steak

7. Peas and carrots

8. Chocolate

9. 6:00 PM

Accuracy (% correct) score _____ %

Speed score _____ minutes

II. PHONE CONVERSATION WITH A FRIEND: RECEIVING A MESSAGE

Directions:

You are going to receive a phone call from a friend. He/she is going to ask you some questions, and you should answer as well as you can. Remember, it is important for you to ask additional questions whenever necessary for clarification.

Write your answers below as well as saying them on the phone.

1. _____

2. _____

3. _____

4. _____

5. _____

6. _____

7. _____

8. _____

9. _____

10. _____

Questions for Open-Set Message: Form A

(Conversant) Hi. I am going to ask some questions.

1. How many people are in your family?

2. Do you have any children?

3. (If #2 is "yes") How many sons?

4. (If #2 is "yes") How many daughters?

5. How old are you now?

6. How old were you when you first started to lose your hearing?

7. Where do you live?

8. Do you drive a car?

9. What kind of car do you have?

10. What is your address?

(Speed dimension is assessed.)

Questions for Open-Set Message: Form B

(Conversant) Hi. I am going to ask some questions.

1. Do you live in a house or an apartment?

2. What is your favorite food?

3. What month comes after August?

4. Where do you go shopping?

5. What is your father's first name?

6. What color is milk?

7. How tall are you?

8. What is your favorite holiday?

9. Are you married or single?

10. What is your telephone number?

(Speed dimension is assessed.)

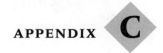

Feelings About Telecommunication

PHONE FORMAT

Please respond to the following statements:

	NA	DS			AS*	

- I know that I can use the telephone to obtain the help I would need in an emergency.   0   1 2 3 4 5
- I have great confidence that the information I obtain over the phone is accurate.   0   1 2 3 4 5
- I enjoy using the telephone to keep in contact with friends and family.   0   1 2 3 4 5
- The telephone is a necessary device in my life.   0   1 2 3 4 5

TDD FORMAT

Please respond to the following statements:

	NA	DS				AS

- I know that I can use the TDD to obtain the help I would need in an emergency.   0   1 2 3 4 5
- I have great confidence that the information I obtain over the TDD is accurate.   0   1 2 3 4 5
- I enjoy using the TDD to keep in contact with friends and family.   0   1 2 3 4 5
- The TDD is a necessary device in my life.   0   1 2 3 4 5

*NA, not applicable; DS, disagree strongly; AS, agree strongly.

CHAPTER 4

Speechreading: Methods and Samples

$\mathbf{T}$HE late-deafened individual who has been recently introduced to an assistive device (i.e., hearing aid, tactile aid, or cochlear implant) must learn to use either an enhanced or completely new receptive modality. The new skills must be compared with prior knowledge and then integrated with the person's existing repertoire to improve communicative ability. Without training in specific skills and strategies for decoding and integrating the new stimuli, the person is at great risk for acquiring incorrect feedback from incomprehensible models.

Although the speechreading literature is extensive, it is largely unhelpful regarding the specifics of training protocols other than to report that rehabilitation is beneficial, to varying degrees, for adults with acquired hearing loss (Rubinstein and Boothroyd, 1987; Pichora-Fuller and Benguerel, 1991). The variation in outcomes reported in the literature may reflect individual professional biases, specific training regimes, and the hearing-impaired individuals themselves, all of which influence success or failure in speechreading training.

Training methods vary widely. Some programs advocate a counseling approach without specific drill, criteria, and goals (Fleming, 1973; Fleming, et al., 1973). However, most speechreading programs are either analytic or synthetic. The analytic programs incorporate training in the discrimination and identification of specific phonemes in a hierarchic fashion in an attempt to improve speechreading skills (Owens, 1978; Smith and Karp, 1978). The synthetic programs stress the whole, rather than specific parts of the speech signal, by using, at a minimum, sentence-length material. Emphasis is placed on obtaining the gist of the message through listening skills, learning of linguistic rules, and situational redundancy (Jeffers and Barley, 1979; Sanders, 1982). Newer teaching techniques stress enhancement of functional communication rather than formal teaching, in order to maximize cues from residual hearing and discourse context (Green and Green, 1984).

One approach may be beneficial for one person but not for another. It is most likely that no one approach is sufficient in and of itself and that a combination of approaches is needed in an integrated and individualized fashion to provide the opportunity for optimal speechreading learning. Based on this rationale, an integrated approach using all methods was developed for our speechreading training protocol.

Specifically, materials and stimuli focusing on behavior modification to improve visual communication, analytic/phoneme level input, synthetic/sentence level input, and integration with residual or new auditory, electrical, or vibrotactile abilities at the conversational level are used. It should be understood that some people will be low-level speechreaders and will require phoneme level skill enhancement but will readily understand the importance of behavioral strategies for speechreading. Therefore more emphasis may be placed on phoneme recognition, followed by overall decoding at the sentence and conversational speech levels, rather than management of situational cues associated with speechreading.

ANALYTIC AND SYNTHETIC DRILL

Analytic and synthetic speechreading skill learning and drill work should be taught in tandem. Requisite baseline analytic skills are needed as groundwork support for synthetic speechreading skills and integration of higher linguistic decoding of the speech message. As will be seen, the simultaneous use of analytic and synthetic speechreading skills along with behavior modification, counseling, and speechtracking techniques can be implemented to achieve the overall goal of enhanced communicative functioning via speechreading.

The profoundly hearing-impaired adult living in and interacting with the hearing world relies heavily on speechreading for correct interpretation of oral discourse (O'Neill and Oyer, 1981). The limits of information transfer achieved, however, by decoding the visual/auditory signal have been well documented. Jeffers and Barley (1980) divided the consonants and vowels into four different visemic (grouping of phonemes by their visual cues) categories. The consonant categories are (1) /p,b,m/; (2) /w,r/; (3) /f,v/; and (4) /θ,ð/, /ʃ,ʒ,tʃ,dʒ/, /s,z/, /t,d,n,l/, and /k,g,ŋ, j/. (Group 4 consonants can be further distinguished by subgroupings.) The vowel categories are (1) /u,ʊ,oʊ,ɤ/; (2) /ɑ,u/; (3) /ɔ,ɔɪ/; and (4) /i,ɪ,eɪ,ʌ,ɛ,æ,a,aɪ. It is easier to identify consonants and vowels across visemic categories than within visemic categories, but, even in the best of conditions, only approximately 70% of speech sounds are interpretable visually. A speaker can produce 13 to 15 speech gestures/second, but the listener's eye can resolve only 8 to 9 gestures/second (McCarthy and Culpepper, 1987). To make the act of speechreading even more difficult, consonant and vowel visual confusions are influenced by speechreading skill, the speaker, positioning and lighting, co-articulation, and rate of speech.

Certain phonemes are more easily identified visually and others more easily identified auditorily. For example, manner of articulation and the voiced/voiceless contrast are more auditorily oriented, while place of articulation is more visually oriented (Miller and Nicely, 1955; Binnie, Jackson, and Montgomery, 1976; Jackson, Montgomery, and Binnie, 1976). The patient must be trained to identify the salient features, whether they are the visual, auditory, or tactile signatures, of the phoneme in order to enhance speechreading skills. In other words, the late-deafened adult must be taught the correct identification of consonants and vowels by either visual and auditory input cues, visual and tactile input cues, or visual and electrical input cues. This provides the speechreader with the requisite information from which to integrate knowledge of individual phonemes for discrimination and decoding of syllables, words, and sentence-length material. These findings relate well to Edgerton's (1985) described later in this chapter.

As part of our clinical trials, we evaluated the visual and audiovisual reception of distinctive features using the Diagnostic Rhyme Test (DRT) (Voiers, 1977). Bhagia (1992) summarized the findings of our longitudinal trials. The subjects were patients undergoing cochlear implantation using single-channel (3M/House or 3M Vienna) or multichannel (Nucleus or Utah [Ineraid]) implants. The implantees were examined using the DRT in visual and audiovisual modes prestimulation, at stimulation, and 3- and 6-months poststimulation.

As a group, the subjects' visual perceptions alone did not improve significantly over time. The subjects relied principally on place of articulation in the visual modality. However, in the audiovisual mode, significant improvement for the total DRT was documented when comparing prestimulation to 3- and 6-month poststimulation intervals. The combined effectiveness of audiovisual feature perception over visual input only was most clearly demonstrated in improvement in scores for voicing and nasality, two features that are visually inaccessible. The subjects obtained graveness, compactness, and sibilation features well. Sustention was conveyed relatively poorly. Bhagia (1992) recommended that when working with implant patients at the analytic level, rehabilitation should concentrate on the development of skill in discrimination of speech features.

Following the acquisition of even rudimentary analytic skills, synthetic speechreading training should be instituted. The clinician must expand speechreading training to include verbal and nonverbal information sources (i.e., active listening, situational redundancy, recognition of gestural and facial cues, and observation of environmental cues) to supplement the paucity of solely visual input. This strategy will increase task attention and maintain motivation because not only is the patient learning to identify individual phonemes but is simultaneously decoding the speech signal and coming to the realization of just how powerful a skill speechreading is when used in conjunction with either enhanced residual or new auditory, electrical, or tactile input cues.

Speechreading, therefore, requires the use of both verbal and nonverbal cues. Speechreading proficiency depends on five primary factors related to the speechreader (Jeffers and Barley, 1979; Chermack, 1981). These are (1) visual perceptual proficiency, (2) ability to synthesize information promoting perceptual and conceptual closure, (3) basic cognitive skills, (4) linguistic facility, and (5) individual personality characteristics, such as flexibility in revising tentative decisions and the ability to guess at meanings.

Since the visible cues of speech are so critical and are relied on heavily by the late-deafened adult in decoding the speech signal, why is speechreading training not provided to the majority of people with acquired hearing loss? Possible reasons are (1) rehabilitation emphasis on amplification, (2) speechreading rehabilitation techniques and measures of progress not clearly defined, (3) trained clinicians in short supply, (4) late-deafened individuals not motivated to commit time and money for speechreading training, and (5) third-party reimbursement unavailable for such services (Pichora-Fuller and Benguerel, 1991).

However, when dealing with the profoundly hearing impaired, speechreading should be considered not a luxury but a necessity for their communicative function. This population is heavily reliant on visual information to supplement their inadequate auditory cues. Speechreading training is needed to enhance poor skills and/or to teach the person to use optimally the new or enhanced auditory code provided by the hearing aid, cochlear implant, or tactile aid.

CASE STUDY 4.1

D.D. was first seen for evaluation in June, 1985. He was 66 years old. His hearing impairment could be dated to an extended hospitalization from 1949-1951 for treatment of tuberculosis, during which he received streptomycin and other potentially ototoxic medications. During his military service, D.D. experienced many physical injuries, especially multiple wounds on the left side of his body.

When D.D. entered our Cochlear Implant Program, he was wearing binaural body hearing aids issued at another VA Medical Center. He communicated poorly, with poor or no lipreading skills. He was not visually attentive and was heavily reliant on written exchanges.

Audiometric assessment found bilateral profound sensorineural hearing loss, with three-frequency pure-tone averages of 108 dB (right) and 106 dB (left) Hearing Level (HL). Spondee thresholds were 92 dB HL (right) and 86 dB HL (left). Aided thresholds yielded a three-frequency average of 63 db Sound Pressure Level (SPL) using the patient's body aids; comparable aided thresholds were obtained using powerful binaural behind-the-ear aids. The patient, therefore, was fit with the latter arrangement.

Baseline evaluation of speechreading using the West Haven Battery (Spitzer et al., 1987) was carried out (Table 4-1). Intensive training was undertaken with the following goals:

- *To increase visual attentiveness*
- *To increase understanding of the speechreading process*
- *To gain skill in speechreading both for short communications and in conversation*

D.D. was considered low functioning in this dimension and required an intensive program, initiated at our center and followed up at his local facility. Table 4-1 shows his follow-up performance after 1 year. The table clearly shows that, after training, there was an improvement in the vision-only category, and, as we would desire, a greater improvement in the combined input category (in this case, vision plus enhanced auditory).

PREPARATION FOR SPEECHREADING: COUNSELING AND FOCUSING ON SKILLS
Behavior Modification

Successful speechreading training incorporates visual input in conjunction with other sensory information (i.e., enhanced auditory, tactile, or electrical cues). The individual must be motivated and have adequate cognitive functioning in order to guess at meanings and integrate disjointed decoded words into a comprehensible message. The stimuli must be graded in rehabilitative difficulty to promote initial and continuing success.

Many late-deafened adults resist speechreading training. Whether their hearing loss was gradual over a long period of time or rapid in onset with fast deterioration, this population remains isolated from mainstream rehabilitative services. They are usually failed hearing aid users or people who have been told that hearing aids would be of no benefit and are either hesitant to try new technology, ignorant of advances, or have given up on any type of assistive device. The consequences are isolation, anger, poor communicative ability, and reliance on a significant other (spouse, friend, or relative) to "speak and hear" for them with

TABLE 4-1 Summary of speechreading performance of D.D. (% correct)

Test	Initial test	Re-test after training	
		Vision only	Vision + assistive device
NAL-West Haven	12	24	46
Iowa-Keaster (Forms A and B)	14	35	70
CID Sentences	0-4	7-20 (Lists A-E)	12-30 (Lists G-H)
Gold Rush Paragraph	0	0	0

the concomitant humiliation, miscommunication, and dependency inherent in this mode of communication.

Late-deafened adults must be counseled in order to change their attitudes and expectations regarding the advanced technology now available: hearing aids, cochlear implants, and vibrotactile devices. The advantages and disadvantages of the technologies need to be explained. The critically important role late-deafened adults play in the rehabilitative process must be stressed. They *are* the most important component in the rehabilitation triad: late-deafened adult—appropriate assistive device—rehabilitation specialist.

Once the late-deafened adult understands, in a global sense, rehabilitation goals and the achievement process, it is important to break the larger issues down into components that the person can more readily understand conceptually and start working toward. Based on individual strengths and weaknesses, initiation and progression through the complex rehabilitation process begins. The late-deafened adult should understand the capabilities and limitations of the individually selected assistive device, the hierarchical steps that will be used to maximize device benefit, and the individualized rehabilitation stimuli that must be reacquired with the new visual and either enhanced auditory, electrical, or vibrotactile input cues.

The overall goal is to achieve a gestalt of (1) correct analytic speechreading skills (by decoding of individual speech components such as phoneme recognition), (2) proper visual attentiveness (by becoming aware of nonlinguistic cues such as facial expression and gestures), (3) manipulation of environmental influences to enhance visual input (by optimal seating, position relative to the speaker, and lighting), (4) auditory input (by decreasing background noise and reverberation) in conjunction with (5) synthetic speechreading skill enhancement (by guessing at and filling in of incomplete parts of the intended message) in order to decode the incoming communicative signal optimally.

Strategic Speechreading and Listening Skills

Strategic listening skills are taught to the late-deafened adult in order that the skills can be employed in conversational situations if the gestalt described previously does not result in satisfactory communication. One such strategic listening skill is employing repair strategies (Tye-Murray, 1991). The strategies used are to (1) repeat the sentence, (2) simplify the sentence, (3) rephrase the sentence, (4) say an important key word, or (5) speak in two sentences. It was found that subjects changed their repair strategies following therapy (i.e., they used the repeat strategy less often and other strategies more often), thereby improving their communicative success.

The final goal is to have the person integrate all inputs to maximize communicative ability. By doing this, each person can stress individual strengths for optimal communicative ability that were learned or enhanced during the rehabilitation process. Implicit in our speechreading program is the individualized nature of rehabilitation. It is most important to expose the person to all the different input modalities and have the best combination adopted for the individual.

Success is a relative term. Success for one person will not be the same for another. Many variables involved in the late-deafened person's hearing loss, communicative functioning, and psychologic profile will determine individual criteria for success. Any improvement in communicative functioning following proper fitting with a device and individualized speechreading training can be viewed as a mark of success.

Speechtracking

The speechtracking procedure used to enhance speechreading skills developed by DeFilippo and Scott (1978) involves a talker, who reads from a prepared text, and a listener, who faces the talker and whose task it is to repeat verbatim the read material. The talker does not continue until each segment is repeated. If the receiver does not repeat the message verbatim, repair strategies may be used by the sender—for example, repeating or rephrasing, emphasizing a key word, using hand gestures, and changing message length (Tye-Murray and Tyler, 1988).

Other researchers have used different repair strategies. Robbins et al. (1985) used a hierarchy of repair strategies in a specific order (i.e., when communication breaks down the sender first repeats the phrase, then rewords it, provides a topic cue, etc. until the message is either understood or the target word is signed or fingerspelled). Owens and Raggio (1987) have a list of repair strategies and the receiver tells the sender which one to use.

Tye-Murray and Tyler (1988) have also shown that speechtracking is beneficial in teaching synthetic and analytic speechreading skills. For example, in synthetic speechreading practice, the receiver can concentrate on overall meanings and key words and not repeat verbatim. In analytic speechreading practice the receiver can repeat every word, as required in the original tracking procedure (DeFilippo and Scott, 1978). A summary of the performance of our patient pool with speechtracking, in quartile ranges, appears in Table 4-2.

Speechtracking is most often used with enhanced auditory (hearing aids) and electrical (cochlear implant) input. Speechtracking, however, has also been used with vibrotactile assistive devices (Cholewiak and Sherrick, 1986). The speaker in that study was multilingual, and, in every instance, speechreading improved with the use of the vibrotactile aid.

It must be mentioned that speechtracking should not be used as a testing method to assess speechreading learning because speechtracking does not reliably measure a person's ability to decode speech (Tye-Murray and Tyler, 1988). For example, when speechreading improves it is not known if the actual skill is im-

TABLE 4-2   Summary of speechtracking performance: quartile ranges (words/min) (N = 31)

Test	$\overline{X}$	SD	Percentile (25th)	Percentile (75th)
Ceiling	18.29	11.46	7	28
Base	3.48	3.42	0	7
Tracking—vision alone	22.35	14.12	16	30
Tracking—vision + hearing aid	27.50	32.68	4	29
Tracking—vision + tactile aid	12.92	24.24	0	14

proving, if the person is more familiar with the sender's facial movements, or if the person has learned better strategies for decoding the message.

METHODS OF ASSESSMENT

The overall goal of our training is to have the person integrate at least one additional sensory input in addition to the visual modality (i.e., enhanced auditory, electrical, or tactile stimulation) for optimal communication. It is felt that visual input with at least one other input modality that is useful for the person's communicative processing and functioning will improve speechreading skills and overall communicative functioning.

Initial evaluation and continuing reassessment during rehabilitation are essential to determine progress in the learning of speechreading skills. The difficulty level of the material is critical and should not exceed a particular individual's experiential or reading background abilities.

A battery of tests for assessment of profoundly hearing-impaired persons was developed at the University of Iowa (Tyler, Preece, and Lowder, 1983). The tests include a number of auditory tests (e.g., Iowa Everyday Sound Recognition) as well as videotaped tests for speechreading assessment. The two most widely used videotapes are (1) Sentence Without Context Test and (2) the Iowa Medial Consonant Sound Test.

The Sentence Without Context Test is a series of low redundancy natural sentences. The Medial Consonant Test assesses the perception of several consonants (i.e., /b,k,ʃ,dʒ,d,m,t,f,n,v,g,p,z,j,s/) in a vowel-consonant-vowel (VCV) context. Each of these tests may be presented as vision-only, vision plus assistive device, or assistive device only.

In addition to these tests, four-color audiovisual speechreading tapes ranging in task difficulty were standardized (Spitzer et al., 1987). The tests were (1) NAL/

West Haven (Appendix A, modified from Plant and Macrase, 1981); (2) Iowa-Keaster, Forms A and B (Appendix B, from Jeffers and Barley, 1971); (3) CID Everyday Sentences (Appendix C, from Davis and Silverman, 1978); and (4) Gold Rush Paragraph (Appendix D, from Schuell, 1965). The hierarchy of responses ranged from answers to questions with the topic known, to verbatim repetition, to abstraction of information from a spoken paragraph in order to answer questions. A range of difficulty was necessary to stress-test good speechreaders and to limit ceiling and floor effects from subjects who would score very well or very poorly if the CID Everyday Sentences were the only speechreading test used.

The order of test difficulty, from easiest to most difficult, is (1) NAL/West Haven, with topics provided and scoring of answers to questions; (2) Iowa-Keaster, Forms A and B, with verbatim responses; (3) CID Everyday Sentences, with key word scoring; and (4) Gold Rush Paragraph, with unfamiliar topic and responding to specific information contained therein. The performance of our subject sample is shown in Table 4-3.

A test battery for assessment of speechreading may include the tests described in Table 4-3 and/or those developed at the University of Iowa (Tyler et al., 1983). These formal tests can be used to determine the person's individual strengths and weaknesses in a controlled environment. They can indicate strategies used by the person (i.e., fixating on one missed word so that the rest of the utterance is missed, tendency to be more successful in speechreading one part of an utterance [beginning, middle, end], the effect of sentence length on accuracy, willingness to attempt to guess the message, and ability to use closure to logically complete the message). Formal assessment should always be supplemented with informal observations of the individual's performance in real-life conversational speech situations because this is the ultimate testing ground.

TABLE 4-3   Speechreading performance on the West Haven Battery (correct responses)

				Quartile cut-off	
Test	N	$\overline{X}$	SD	25th	75th
NAL-West Haven	33	20.42	11.52	10	29
CID Sentences	29	112.90	89.12	28	169
Iowa-Keaster (Form A)	17	64.00	51.26	22	94.5
Iowa-Keaster (Form B)	16	82.94	51.22	35	125
Gold Rush Paragraph	31	1.04	1.53	0	1

EXPECTATIONS OF PERFORMANCE

Formal test results and informal observations will suggest the starting point for training. Training should be initiated one objective lower than suggested by the evaluation to ensure initial experience of success. As each criterion is met, more challenging goals are introduced. If the person reaches a plateau, branching to slightly easier material should be undertaken until progress can occur.

We developed a pragmatic approach to selection and presentation of stimuli. Such an approach is more accessible to use by clinicians who do not have access to or use of expensive equipment such as video laser discs. Speechreading training should always be conducted using normal speech patterns of intensity, rate, pitch, intonation, and voicing. It is not recommended that stimuli be presented unvoiced because eliminating voicing creates an unnatural communication environment, alters articulatory movements, and, most importantly, does not allow for multimodality input (i.e., the person's use of the selected assistive device).

HOW TO USE THE SPEECHREADING TRAINING MATERIALS

The stimuli used in this chapter are only suggestions. Counseling concerning assistive devices does not vary significantly from person to person (Rubenstein and Boothroyd, 1987). Analytic rehabilitation stimuli are also not very variable across late-deafened individuals, and the synthetic sentence and discourse level goals follow the same general hierarchy regardless of the input modality and device employed. However, the basic phoneme differential skills that need to be acquired are specific to the assistive device the person uses (see Edgerton, 1985, for a comprehensive distinctive feature approach to phoneme identification with cochlear implants).

The differences in rehabilitation are mainly centered on the rate of advancement through the hierarchy of speechreading acquisition steps. Some late-deafened individuals will progress rapidly and others much more slowly. The most important aspects of training are the individualized nature of the rehabilitation and the importance of maintaining motivation and success levels. The actual stimuli used should be geared to the individual patient's interests and needs whenever possible.

It is hoped that individualized stimuli geared to the person's areas of interest will be used in order to maintain interest and motivation level. Areas to keep in mind are daily living skills, overlearned phrases, hobbies, and occupational terms. The earliest and easiest stimuli should be loaded with visual cues for easy identification of target phonemes, words, and sentences. As progress is made, objectives should shift to overall communicative ability by incorporating linguistic and non linguistic cues and topic areas that are both known and unknown to the speechreader.

It is important to remember that this chapter is designed as a tool to enhance and improve the late-deafened person's overall communicative ability and, as such, it should be used in its entirety. No single part should be used in isolation, as it is the philosophy of this manual that an integrated holistic approach to speechreading training is required for optimal learning and success.

THERAPY PLANS: GOALS, OBJECTIVES, AND SUCCESS CRITERIA

I. Communication Strategies

A. GOAL: To *effect* the use of supplementary nonauditory communication strategies into the overall communication process:

    a. Nonauditory visual cues—lip movements, facial expressions, gestures

    b. Assertiveness training—manipulating the environment (situational cues, topic being discussed)

    c. Assertiveness training—response to auditory failure (skills needed to change failure into success)

All strategies lead to increased reception of communicative intent. Once discussion of the strategies has been completed, the demonstration of such cues should be employed. Role playing and homework assignments help to accomplish this task. It is important to keep the task topical and pertinent to each patient.

    1. Objective: To *understand* the importance of nonauditory (i.e., visual cues) in the overall communication process.

    Procedure: Discuss the various nonauditory visual cues available for use during the communication process—specifically (a) lip movements, (b) facial expressions, and (c) gestures.

    Criterion: Clinician monitoring—90% success rate.

                Self-monitoring—90% success rate.

    Materials: Role-playing examples:

    a. Two people sit back-to-back and carry on a conversation. After the conversation they and the clinician discuss what happened. Then the same pair face one another and have the same conversation. The discussion that follows should focus on the contribution of visual cues to the communication process.

    b. Two people have a conversation under two different conditions. First, they use minimal visual cues (minimum lip movements, facial expressions, no gestures, etc.). Second, the natural, not exaggerated, visual cues are incorporated into the conversation. The discussion that follows will highlight the importance of watching the speaker closely, especially the lips and face.

B. GOAL: To *create* awareness and *implement* assertive behavior

1. **Objective:** To *understand* the importance of assertiveness training—specifically (a) manipulating the environment by enhancing situational cues and (b) having knowledge of the topic being discussed in the overall communication process.

   Procedure: Discuss the various means available to manipulate the environment (Appendix E). Be sure to include:

   a. Establishing a noise-free environment (i.e., requesting that background music be lowered/turned off, closing doors, requesting rooms with good acoustics).

   b. Procuring the most advantageous position relative to the speaker (i.e., arriving early for best seating options and sitting up front to hear and see better).

   c. Correcting poor lighting situations so that the speaker is clearly visible (i.e., not having the light directly behind the speaker and shining into your eyes).

   d. Observing participants' movements and reactions and making suggestions (i.e., requesting speakers to sit in selected positions for optimal visual input).

   e. Promoting one-on-one conversations rather than group discussions, when possible.

   Criterion: Clinician monitoring—90% success rate.

   Self-monitoring—90% success rate.

   Materials: Role playing, using the previous examples as guides for situations (see Objective 1, Goal A). Assign homework requiring a list of ways the individual has manipulated the environment effectively. Observe a group situation in which all of the previously discussed environmental factors have been unstructured and list ways to use successfully the learned techniques in such situations.

2. **Objective:** To *understand* the importance of assertiveness training—specifically, response to auditory failure—in the overall communication process. The person must respond promptly to an auditory failure. If such a failure is not corrected quickly by having the person ask for a repetition or clarification of the misunderstood point, a problem will arise because of subsequent misunderstanding regarding what the conversation is about (Giolas, 1982). The late-deafened person must develop a repertoire of responses to auditory failure.

   Procedure: Discuss the various ways to respond to auditory failure. Be sure to include:

   a. Requesting repetition of a missed message and repeating the part heard to facilitate conversational flow.

b. Adjusting volume of amplification device depending on the loudness of different speakers.

c. Admitting having a hearing impairment and telling the speaker the most successful way to have two-way communication.

d. Asking significant others to fill in pieces of a missing message when you are unable to interrupt speaker or the topic of the conversation has changed.

e. Stressing the importance of guessing and attempting to follow the discussion despite missing some information (i.e., often gestural or situational cues will help get you back on track).

f. Trying not to pretend you understand because it will create more difficulty later in the conversation.

g. Focusing on ideas rather than isolated words.

Criterion: Self-monitoring—90% success rate.

Clinician monitoring—90% success rate.

Materials: Role playing using the previous guidelines for situations. Assign homework requiring listing instances of how persons respond to auditory failure.

3. **Objective:** To *combine* and *integrate* the information and skills acquired in Objectives 1 and 2.

Procedure: To employ tasks that will provide opportunity to effectively integrate the nonauditory strategies for optimal communication.

Criterion: Self-monitoring—90% success rate.

Clinician monitoring—90% success rate.

Materials: Such tasks can include homework assignments that require discussion of a particular newspaper article or sporting event, role playing, or a trip to the shopping mall, hospital, store, and/or cafeteria with the particular goal of acquiring certain information.

A more specific response to auditory failure (i.e., a five-step repair strategy [Tye-Murray, 1991]) is taught to increase communication success. Specifically, the hearing-impaired individual will be aware of and be able to use the repair strategy or strategies best suited to maximizing understanding. The steps are repetition of the entire sentence, simplification of the sentence, rephrasing of the sentence, saying an important key word from the sentence, or speaking in two separate sentences. For example:

Repair strategy	Example
Primary:	The dog is eating the food.
Rephrase:	The dog is hungry.
Simplify:	The dog eats.
Key word:	Eats
Two sentences:	The dog is hungry. The dog is eating.

II. Training in speech reading: phonemes, words, sentences, and conversation

A. GOAL: To *integrate* visual + assistive device (visual + auditory; visual + electrical; or visual + vibrotactile) inputs for purposes of efficient phoneme identification.

    1. Objective: To *teach* perception of the distinctive features of place of production, manner of production, and voicing for the English phonemes, following the distinctive feature hierarchy described by Edgerton (1985) (see box below).

    Procedure: The listener should use visual + assistive device cues to learn the individual characteristic visual and acoustic/tactile signatures of the phonemes. Examples are provided of each category of phoneme. The words are not arranged in ascending order of difficulty and the clinician can use any combination of phoneme blocks. The patient is permitted to read the stimuli in conjunction with enhanced auditory, electrical, or vibrotactile input in order to learn the specific signature of the assistive device used.

    Criterion: Clinician monitoring—90% success rate.

CONSONANT FEATURE HIERARCHY FROM EASY TO DIFFICULT FOR DISCRIMINATION TRAINING WITH RHYMING AND NONRHYMING WORD PAIRS

Initial consonant contrasts

1. Unvoiced plosive vs. Voiced continuant
2. Voiced plosive vs. Voiced continuant
3. Voiced continuant vs. Unvoiced continuant
4. Unvoiced plosive vs. Unvoiced continuant
5. Voiced plosive vs. Unvoiced plosive
6. Voiced plosive vs. Unvoiced continuant

Final consonant contrasts

1. Unvoiced plosive vs. Voiced continuant
2. Voiced plosive vs. Voiced continuant
3. Voiced continuant vs. Unvoiced continuant
4. Unvoiced plosive vs. Unvoiced continuant
5. Voiced plosive vs. Unvoiced plosive
6. Voiced plosive vs. Unvoiced continuant

From Edgerton BJ: *Semin Hear* 6:65-90, 1985.

Materials:

INITIAL CONSONANT CONTRASTS

1. Unvoiced Plosive   vs.   Voiced Continuant

/p/	/m/
pop	mom
paid	made
pail	mail
pay	may
pound	mound
pepper	mommy
paper	maybe
piper	matter
popper	meter
puppet	mugger

/t/	/n/
tot	not
tame	name
tip	nip
tune	noon
take	neck
taper	neighbor
token	noodle
tiger	napkin
tiptoe	nighttime
tepid	notice

/k/	/l/
cake	lake
cook	look
corn	learn
can	lamb
cot	lot
cookie	looking
candy	lettuce
couple	luggage
cupboard	landed
candle	ladle

Objective 2, follows on p. 125.

2. Voiced Plosive   vs.   Voiced Continuant

/b/	/m/
bake	make
beet	meet
bet	met
bought	mop
bale	mail
baby	maybe
baboon	miner
banner	manner
ballot	mallet
begin	metal
batter	matter

/d/	/n/
dog	nod
deck	neck
dock	knock
dig	nick
doll	knoll
dagger	notice
data	never
dizzy	noisy
duty	naughty
dapper	neuter

/g/	/l/
got	lot
give	live
gone	lawn
gold	load
game	lame
garden	leather
garlic	lilac
gopher	loafer
gateway	locker
gavel	later

3. Voiced Continuant   vs.   Unvoiced Continuant

/v/	**/f/**
vile	file
vice	fife
vet	fat
vale	fail
veal	feel
viper	fiber
value	follow
veto	fatal
vigor	figure
viking	fickle

/z/	**/s/**
zoo	sue
zap	sap
zeal	seal
zag	sag
zoom	soon
zipper	summer
zebra	soccer
zoning	setting
zigzag	sagging
zippy	simmer

/m/	**/ʃ/**
mum	shun
mine	shine
moo	shoe
mock	shock
mime	ship
monkey	shampoo
money	shipshape
mudhole	showtime
measure	shower
mailman	shimmer

/ð/
the
they
this
then
there
themselves
therefore
thereby
The Bronx
The Times

/θ/
thick
thaw
thank
thin
thought
thumbnail
thinking
thunder
Thursday
thimble

4. Unvoiced Plosive   vs.   Unvoiced Continuant

/p/
poke
pick
pool
pine
pole
padlock
parking
pigpen
pillow
peanut

/f/
folk
fit
fool
fine
fold
football
footprint
famous
fellow
phantom

/t/
tent
time
tune
tone
tip
target
tennis
toilet
Tuesday
tightrope

/s/
sent
sing
soon
song
sip
sargent
senate
sonnet
someday
songbird

/k/

corn

cuff

court

kook

kiss

cargo

cocktail

cobweb

cocoa

confirm

/ʃ/

shown

shove

short

shoot

ship

sharpen

shirttail

shortbread

shortcut

shopping

5. Voiced Plosive   vs.   Unvoiced Plosive

/b/

base

beach

bath

bear

bill

beeline

before

because

bikepath

boxcar

/p/

pace

peach

path

pear

pill

peapod

pencil

perform

pigeon

popcorn

/d/

dime

doe

dame

dart

doom

daisy

dealer

dollar

downtown

dumbbell

/t/

time

toe

tame

tart

tomb

tackle

tender

taller

topsoil

toothpick

/g/	/k/
guide	cord
gone	coin
goof	cough
gum	come
gown	cow
goodbye	cowboy
gopher	coffee
guilty	confess
guppy	cutting
gimmick	comic

6. Voiced Plosive   vs.   Unvoiced continuant

/b/	/s/
bay	say
bye	sigh
beg	said
bike	side
bun	sun
baker	sicker
batter	sadder
beetle	saddle
bouquet	socket
building	songbird

/d/	/f/
dense	fence
dill	fill
dine	fine
do	few
done	fun
doorstop	foretold
downhill	farmhouse
doorknob	forgive
doubtful	foolish
depart	female

/g/

gum
girl
goal
gas
gulp
goldfish
gaslight
gimmick
gather
guidebook

/b,d,g/

bass
bean
beep
dock
dove
door
go
good
gave
bedspread
backbone
bedbug
dog pound
dollhouse
doorman
gazelle
gallop
gumdrop

/θ/

thumb
thirst
thud
thanks
thump
thoughtful
thankless
thimble
thirteen
thighbone

/ʃ/

shack
sheen
sheep
shock
shove
shore
show
should
shave
sheepskin
shipboard
shampoo
shotgun
showroom
sureshot
shadow
shallow
showman

FINAL CONSONANT CONTRASTS

1. Unvoiced Plosive   vs.   Voiced Continuant

/p/	**/m/**
top	Tom
hop	home
type	time
soap	some
cop	comb
turnip	twosome
cleanup	condemn
backup	bathroom
pushup	problem
mousetrap	moonbeam
/t/	**/n/**
pit	pin
suit	soon
but	bun
beat	been
sit	sin
checkmate	chowmein
footnote	foreseen
pollute	pipeline
remote	ravine
walnut	wagon
/k/	**/l/**
walk	wall
pack	pail
week	wheel
tick	tail
joke	jail
outlook	oatmeal
cookbook	footstool
fullback	football
sidewalk	payroll
headache	topsoil

2. Voiced Plosive   vs.   Voiced Continuant

/b/	**/m/**
Bob	bomb
tube	tomb
mob	home
cube	comb
lab	home
bathtub	boredom
bathrobe	moonbeam
earlobe	extreme
doorknob	daytime
ice cube	ice cream

/d/	**/n/**
mad	man
sad	Sam
time	tin
bead	seen
read	ran
fishfood	fireman
rye bread	goosedown
plywood	postpone
railroad	shoeshine
seaweed	soybean

/g/	**/l/**
dog	doll
hog	hall
pig	pill
mug	mill
sag	sail
hot dog	eggshell
icebag	high school
eggnog	Knob Hill
dog tag	mothball
nutmeg	seashell

3. Voiced Continuant   vs.   Unvoiced Continuant

/m/	**/s/**
team	miss
some	peace
rhyme	rice
name	nice
calm	kiss
custom	confess
bottom	address
became	bookcase
random	racehorse
mushroom	shameless
/n/	**/f/**
seen	beef
tan	safe
pin	leaf
done	tough
run	roof
common	enough
mountain	housewife
trombone	rainproof
thirteen	takeoff
homerun	layoff
/l/	**/θ/**
pail	path
tool	tooth
mail	math
call	moth
bill	myth
tumble	mammoth
mouthful	blacksmith
oatmeal	beneath
pigtail	locksmith
beachball	Babe Ruth

/m,n,l/	/ʃ/
hum	hush
tame	sash
calm	cash
ban	bash
win	wish
bone	dish
fill	fish
tale	dash
whale	wash
pull	push
redeem	radish
sunbeam	rubbish
twosome	toothbrush
chicken	childish
common	catfish
fortune	foolish
faithful	furnish
downfall	nailbrush
pinwheel	polish
seashell	selfish

4. Unvoiced Plosive   vs.   **Unvoiced Contintuant**

/p/	/s/
leap	less
chop	toss
peep	peace
deep	dice
lip	loose
roundtrip	Paris
shipshape	shapeless
windpipe	wordless
housetop	shoelace
jumprope	police

/t/	/f/
hate	half
met	deaf
cot	cough
cheat	chief
write	wife
minute	relief
sailboat	jackknife
wallet	showoff
flashlight	fireproof
donut	dandruff

/k/	/θ/
sock	south
weak	wrath
cake	faith
beak	teeth
bike	wreath
cheesecake	steambath
bike rack	goldsmith
notebook	phone booth
public	Plymouth
technique	untruth

/**p,t,k**/
up
whip
shape
bait
jot
classmate
broomstick
clambake
headache
earthquake

/**ʃ**/
bush
wash
crash
trash
josh
toothbrush
whitewash
relish
sheepish
eyelash

5. Voiced Plosive vs. Unvoiced Plosive

/**b**/
hob
babe
knob
tub
web
sparerib
health club
bathrobe
earlobe
prescribe

/**p**/
hop
tape
nope
top
wipe
skislope
pet shop
cough drop
landscape
peace pipe

/**d**/
toad
wade
road
dad
feed
flash flood
concede
decode
succeed
railroad

/**t**/
toot
wait
write
date
feet
dropout
conceit
delight
repeat
showboat

/g/	**/k/**
bug	buck
leg	lake
sag	sack
rug	reek
wig	week
bedbug	backache
fatigue	cupcake
shoe bag	deadlock
jet lag	lunch break
shag rug	livestock

6. Voiced Plosive   vs.   Unvoiced Continuant

/b/	**/s/**
gab	gas
sob	us
robe	boss
rob	toss
tube	yes
wolf cub	greenhouse
skylab	nervous
corncob	townhouse
backrub	porpoise
cobweb	Kansas

/d/	**/f/**
add	half
load	loaf
fried	knife
read	rough
wide	safe
avoid	belief
beside	giraffe
firewood	penknife
prepaid	fire chief
seafood	sunroof

/g/

dog
rag
vague
fog
dig
time lag
sandbag
teabag
zigzag
hedgehog

/b,d,g/

knob
sub
rib
fad
rod
dead
bag
mug
wag
fig
adlib
ice cube
yacht club
flash flood
seaweed
postpaid
ice bag
bigwig
spark plug
shindig

/θ/

death
wreath
warmth
faith
fourth
untruth
sunbath
flight path
sabbath
sweet tooth

/ʃ/

nosh
cash
rush
fish
rash
dish
bash
mush
lush
mash
carwash
cod fish
foolish
mouthwash
starfish
paintbrush
Irish
backlash
publish
Spanish

2. **Objective:** To *discriminate* the distinctive features of place of production, manner of production, and voicing for the English phonemes following the hierarchy described by Edgerton (1985).

   Procedure: The listener should use visual + assistive device cues to discriminate the signatures of the phoneme pairs.

   Criterion: Clinician monitoring—90% success rate.

Materials:

INITIAL CONSONANT CONTRASTS

1. Unvoiced Plosive   vs.   Voiced Continuant

/p/	/m/
pound	mound
paper	maybe
popper	meter
puppet	mugger
paid	maid
pop	mom
pay	may
pepper	mommy
pail	mail

/t/	/n/
taper	neighbor
tepid	notice
tot	not
tip	nip
take	neck
tiger	napkin
tune	noon
tame	name
tiptoe	nighttime
token	noodle

/k/	/l/
can	lamb
couple	luggage
candle	ladle
cake	lake
cookie	looking
cupboard	landed
candy	lettuce
cot	lot
cook	look
corn	learn

2. Voiced Plosive   vs.   Voiced Continuant

/b/	/m/
baboon	miner
bale	male
beet	meet
batter	matter
ballot	mallet
begin	metal
banner	manner
bake	make
bought	mop
baby	maybe
bet	met

/d/	/n/
dagger	notice
data	never
dapper	neuter
dog	nod
doll	knoll
duty	naughty
deck	neck
dizzy	noisy
dock	not
dig	nick

/g/	/l/
gateway	locker
gavel	later
garden	leather
gone	lawn
got	lot
garlic	lilac
gold	load
gopher	loafer
give	live
game	lame

3. Voiced Continuant   vs.   Unvoiced Continuant

/v/	/f/
value	follow
vigor	figure
viking	fickle
vale	fail
veal	feel
vice	fife
veto	fatal
viper	fiber
vile	file
vet	fat

/z/	/s/
zoom	soon
zeal	seal
zippy	simmer
zap	sap
zebra	soccer
zoo	sue
zoning	setting
zag	sag
zipper	summer
zigzag	sagging

/m/	/ʃ/
mailman	shimmer
mudhole	showtime
monkey	shampoo
mock	shock
mine	shine
money	shipshape
measure	shower
mum	shun
mime	ship
moo	shoe

/ð/

this
therefore
The Times
then
The Bronx
the
there
themselves
they
thereby

/θ/

thank
thinking
thimble
thin
Thursday
thick
thought
thumbnail
thaw
thunder

4. Unvoiced Plosive   vs.   Unvoiced continuant

/p/

pigpen
pine
poke
parking
peanut
pool
pillow
pick
padlock
pole

/f/

famous
fine
folk
footprint
phantom
fool
fellow
fit
football
fold

/t/

tennis
Tuesday
tent
toilet
tone
tip
tightrope
tune
time
target

/s/

senate
Sunday
sent
sonnet
song
sip
songbird
soon
same
sargent

/k/	/ʃ/
cocoa	shortcut
kiss	ship
cargo	sharpen
confirm	shopping
court	short
cocktail	shirttail
corn	shown
cobweb	shortbread
kook	shoot
cuff	shove

5. Voiced Plosive   vs.   Unvoiced Plosive

/b/	/p/
bikepath	pigeon
beeline	peapod
base	pace
bear	pear
because	perform
boxcar	popcorn
bill	pill
beach	peach
bath	path
before	pencil

/d/	/t/
dealer	tender
doom	tomb
dime	time
downtown	topsoil
dart	tart
dumbbell	toothpick
daisy	tackle
dame	tame
dollar	taller
doe	toe

/g/	**/k/**
goof	cough
guilty	confess
gown	cow
guide	cord
gone	coin
gopher	coffee
gimmick	comic
guppy	cutting
gum	come
goodbye	cowboy

6. Voiced Plosive   vs.   Unvoiced Continuant

/b/	**/s/**
bouquet	socket
bay	say
bun	sun
building	songbird
batter	sadder
bye	sigh
beetle	saddle
baker	sicker
bike	side
beg	said

/d/	**/f/**
done	fun
depart	female
dense	fence
do	few
dine	fine
doubtful	foolish
doorknob	forgive
doorstop	foretold
dill	fill
downhill	farmhouse

/g/

gas
girl
guidebook
gaslight
gum
gulp
gimmick
goal
goldfish
gas

/θ/

thanks
thirst
thighbone
thankless
thumb
thump
thimble
thud
thoughtful
thanks

/b,d,g/

beep
bass
bean
dove
door
dock
good
go
gave
bedspread
bedbug
backbone
doorman
dollhouse
dog pound
gallop
gazelle
gumdrop

/ʃ/

sheep
shack
sheen
shove
shore
shock
should
show
shave
sheepskin
shampoo
shipboard
sureshot
showroom
shotgun
shallow
shadow
showman

FINAL CONSONANT CONTRASTS

1. Unvoiced Plosive   vs.   Voiced Continuant

/p/	**/m/**
type	time
hop	home
turnip	twosome
cop	comb
mousetrap	moonbeam
cleanup	condemn
pushup	problem
top	Tom
backup	bathroom
soap	some

/t/	**/n/**
checkmate	chow mein
walnut	wagon
sit	sin
suit	soon
pollute	pipeline
pit	pin
remote	ravine
beat	been
but	bun
footnote	foreseen

/k/	**/l/**
sidewalk	payroll
tick	tail
headache	topsoil
fullback	football
walk	wall
weak	wheel
cookbook	footstool
pack	pail
outlook	oatmeal
joke	jail

2. Voiced Plosive   vs.   Voiced Continuant

/b/	/m/
earlobe	extreme
lab	home
tube	tomb
bathrobe	moonbeam
Bob	bomb
ice cube	ice cream
mob	home
doorknob	daytime
cube	comb
bathtub	boredom

/d/	/n/
read	ran
time	tim
plywood	postpone
fishfood	fireman
mad	man
seaweed	soybean
railroad	shoeshine
bead	seen
rye bread	goosedown
sad	sam

/g/	/l/
dog	doll
nutmeg	seashell
icebag	high school
pig	pill
sag	sail
hog	hall
dog tag	mothball
mug	mill
eggnog	Knob Hill
hot dog	eggshell

3. Voiced Continuant   vs.   Unvoiced Continuant

/m/	/s/
custom	confess
rhyme	rice
mushroom	shameless
became	bookcase
team	miss
name	nice
random	racehorse
bottom	address
calm	kiss
some	peace

/n/	/f/
done	tough
tan	safe
seen	beef
homerun	layoff
mountain	housewife
thirteen	takeoff
trombone	rainproof
common	enough
run	roof
pin	leaf

/l/	/θ/
mouthful	blacksmith
beachball	Babe Ruth
bill	myth
pail	path
call	moth
pigtail	locksmith
tumble	mammoth
tool	tooth
oatmeal	beneath
male	math

/m,n,l/	/ʃ/
calm	cash
hum	hush
tame	sash
win	wish
ban	bash
bone	dish
tail	dash
whale	wash
pull	push
fill	fish
sunbeam	rubbish
redeem	radish
twosome	toothbrush
common	catfish
fortune	foolish
chicken	childish
pinwheel	Polish
seashell	selfish
faithful	furnish
downfall	nailbrush

4. Unvoiced Plosive   vs.   Unvoiced Continuant

/p/	/s/
lip	loose
peep	peace
chop	toss
deep	dice
leap	less
windpipe	wordless
housetop	shoelace
roundtrip	Paris
jumprope	police
shipshape	shapeless

/t/
cot
cheat
met
minute
flashlight
donut
wallet
sailboat
right
hate

/k/
cake
beak
technique
notebook
bike
weak
bike rack
public
sock
cheesecake

/p,t,k/
jot
whip
shape
up
broomstick
earthquake
classmate
bait
clambake
headache

/f/
cough
chief
deaf
relief
fireproof
dandruff
showoff
jackknife
wife
half

/θ/
faith
teeth
untruth
phone booth
wreath
wrath
goldsmith
Plymouth
south
steambath

/ʃ/
josh
wash
crash
bush
whitewash
eyelash
toothbrush
trash
relish
sheepish

5. Voiced Plosive   vs.   Unvoiced Plosive

/b/	/p/
health club	pet shop
prescribe	peace pipe
tub	top
earlobe	landscape
hob	hop
knob	nope
sparerib	skislope
bathrobe	cough drop
web	wipe
babe	tape

/d/	/t/
flash flood	dropout
decode	delight
wade	wait
feed	feet
railroad	showboat
concede	conceit
rode	right
dad	date
succeed	repeat
toad	toot

/g/	/k/
bedbug	backache
jet lag	lunch break
bug	buck
shoe bag	deadlock
sag	sack
wig	weak
shag rug	livestock
rug	reek
leg	lake
fatigue	cupcake

6. Voiced Plosive   vs.   Unvoiced Continuant

/b/	**/s/**
tube	yes
robe	boss
sob	us
skylab	nervous
cobweb	Kansas
rob	toss
backrub	porpoise
corncob	townhouse
gab	gas
wolf cub	greenhouse

/d/	**/f/**
read	rough
fried	knife
prepaid	fire chief
seafood	sunroof
add	half
beside	giraffe
avoid	belief
firewood	penknife
wide	safe
load	loaf

/g/	**/θ/**
dig	fourth
teabag	flight path
hedgehog	sweet tooth
rag	wreath
sandbag	sunbath
fog	faith
dog	death
vague	warmth
zigzag	sabbath
time lag	untruth

/b,d,g/	/ʃ/
rib	rush
sub	cash
nob	nosh
dead	dish
rod	rash
fad	fish
wag	lush
bag	bash
mug	mush
fig	mash
ice cube	cod fish
yacht club	foolish
adlib	carwash
postpaid	paintbrush
flash flood	mouthwash
seaweed	starfish
shindig	Spanish
spark plug	publish
bigwig	backlash
icebag	Irish

3. **Objective:** To *identify* the phonemes of English following the hierarchy described by Edgerton (1985).

   Procedure: The listener will use visual + assistive device cues to *identify* the target phoneme in a word environment. Instructions are: "We are working on _____ (specific phoneme). You will tell me which sound begins the word. You have in your hand a list of possible choices. Are you ready?"

   The clinician will present a list of 10 words selected on the basis of the criteria suggested by Edgerton (1985). The patient will hold a list of phonemes coordinated to the word. For instance, during a trial for contrasts of plosives vs. continuants, the patient's list may contain /p,b,t,d,k,g,f,v,s,z, θ,δ,m,n,l/, depending on the particular distinctive feature targeted for identification.

   Criterion: Clinician monitoring—90% success rate.

   Materials: Trials will proceed from easier to harder stimuli identifications. Hierarchy is the same as in Table 4-2 and involves initial and final consonant contrasts (see box on p. 110). The clinician may use word lists from Objective 1, Goal A as long as the words are presented in random order. Additional word lists may be generated at the clinician's discretion.

B. **GOAL:** To *integrate* visual + assistive device (visual + auditory; visual + electrical; or visual + vibrotactile) inputs for efficient receptive communication of words, phrases, and sentence-length material with the topic known. NOTE: The clinician can use live voice or stimuli recorded on videotape.

   1. **Objective:** In a quiet therapy situation, to *identify* individual words with the category known to the listener.

      Procedure: The clinician will provide the topic (e.g., baseball). The listener will use visual + assistive device cues. The stimulus word should be embedded within a carrier phrase. Begin with single-syllable words placed at the end of a carrier phrase (e.g., "Here is the _____ ."). Then place the word within the carrier phrase (e.g., "The _____ is here."). At each step, familiarize the listener with the carrier phrase before beginning the therapy trial. Repeat with two- and then three-syllable words. If success is not seen at the initiation of a new step, alternate between the old and the new step. If success is not seen at the beginning of this objective, provide the listener with a closed set, familiarizing him/her with two to five choices for the stimulus item. If success is not achieved at this level, use a present/absent criterion for the stimulus word and work toward increasing complexity. Word lists can be designed to fit the listener's needs and interests, and the carrier phrase can be tailored to fit the stimulus category.

      Criterion: Clinician monitoring—90% success rate.

      Materials: Any appropriate commercially prepared or self-made word and sentence lists used by the clinician to fit the needs and interests of the client. Additional topics can be generated to meet the needs and motivational level of the individual patient.

HIGH VISIBILITY
The topic is baseball.

Here is the bat.
Here is the ball.
Here is the glove.
Here is the base.
Here is the mitt.

The player is here.
The catcher is here.
The field is here.
The dugout is here.
The umpire is here.

The topic is cooking.

Here is the pot.
Here is the food.
Here is the stove.
Here is the spoon.
Here is the sink.

The fork is here.
The salt and pepper are here.
The blender is here.
The meat is here.
The spices are here.

LOW VISIBILITY
The topic is driving.

Here is the car.
Here is the driver.
Here is the highway.
Here is the stop sign.
Here is the brake.

The horn is here.
The truck is here.

The exit is here.
The radio is here.
The map is here.

The topic is work.

Here is the job.
Here is the desk.
Here is the telephone.
Here is the fax machine.
Here is the boss.

The secretary is here.
The lunchroom is here.
The pencil sharpener is here.
The copy machine is here.
The paycheck is here.

2. **Objective:** In a quiet therapy situation, to *comprehend* short sentences of simple structure (i.e., [subject + verb; subject + verb + object]) with the subject known to the listener.

Procedure: The listener will use visual + assistive device cues. Construct sentences that fit the listener's needs and interests. At the initiation of this objective, it is suggested that phoneme articulatory visibility and the individual acoustic/tactile signatures of the phonemes be reviewed. Use repair strategies to elicit correct responses.

Sentences with high visibility loading will be used first, followed by sentences with low visibility loading (i.e., words with bilabial phonemes vs. lingua-alveolar phonemes).

Criterion: Clinician monitoring—90% success rate.

Materials: Any appropriate commercially prepared or self-made word and sentence lists used by the clinician to fit the needs and interests of the client. Additional topics can be generated to meet the needs and motivational level of the individual patient.

HIGH VISIBILITY
The topic is shopping for food.

I like to eat bananas.
I buy food at the market.
I like to eat bread.
Pears and pineapples are fruit.
I spend a lot of money on food.
Peanut butter is my favorite food.

The parking lot at the market is full.
The shopping bag broke.
I buy frozen food.
Pretzels and potato chips are junk food.

The topic is movies.

Most movies cost 5 dollars.
My favorite movie is playing this week.
I like to see the movies.
Most movies are 3 hours.
Monster movies are my favorite.
I buy popcorn at the movies.
The movie was boring.
My friend and I go to the movies.
This is the movie theater.
Movies are always fun.

LOW VISIBILITY
The topic is animals.

My dog has spots.
I don't like cats.
A snake is not a good pet.
My canary died.
The giraffe has a long neck.
Lions and tigers are dangerous.
The zebra has stripes.
Do you like animals?
I have a pet goat.
You can ride a horse.

The topic is hobbies.

Stamp collecting is very rewarding.
Hobbies add much to your life.
Knitting sweaters takes a long time.
Every hobby has a magazine.
Drawing takes a lot of practice.
Coin collecting is expensive.
Hobbies help to make friends.
Everyone should have a hobby.
How do you like your hobby?
I spend 2 hours a day on sewing.

3. **Objective:** In a quiet therapy situation, to *comprehend* longer sentences of increasing complexity of structure (i.e., [subject + verb + object + modifier/dependent clause]) with the subject known to the listener. Sentences with high visibility loading will be used first, followed by sentences with low visibility loading.

   Procedure: Same as Objective 2, Goal B. There are three methods to approach this stage. In the first, the clinician simply tells the listener the subject being discussed. In the second, the clinician reads a paragraph and then asks questions concerning its content. In the third method, the patient speechtracks the paragraph. It is necessary to ask questions regarding content to ensure that the patient has obtained the gist of the paragraph.

   Criterion: Clinician monitoring—90% success rate.

   Materials: Any appropriate commercially prepared or self-made word and sentence lists used by the clinician to fit the needs and interests of the client. Other suggested topics for this type of trial are going on vacation, going to the library, riding a bike, family relationships, playing sports, and current events.

   HIGH VISIBILITY
   The topic is school.

   My father finished high school but went to work later.
   Many boys play football in high school, but they must work very hard to pass their classes.
   The president of the university must be a well-known person.
   My professor teaches math on Monday but not on Friday.
   My classes begin at seven in the morning and they finish by noon.

   LOW VISIBILITY
   The topic is building a house.

   You will have to buy many tools and learn to use them to build a house.
   You should subcontract with a plumber and electrician if you don't have these skills.
   Be sure to follow building codes for your city when you plan your house.
   Interview several contractors before you decide who should build your house.
   An architect can help design the house, but you have the final word on the plan.

4. **Objective:** In a quiet therapy situation, to *comprehend* short sentences of simple structure (i.e., [subject + verb; subject + verb + object]) with the subject *not* known to the listener.

Procedure: The listener will use visual + assistive device cues. Construct sentences that fit the listener's needs and interests. At this stage, the intent is to help the listener achieve communication competence in normal spontaneous social situations. If the listener has difficulty at the outset with this objective, have him/her relate the gist of the conversation rather than word-by-word responses. Verbatim responses are not the goal. Use repair strategies to enhance receptive skills.

Criterion: Clinician monitoring—90% success rate.

Materials: Any appropriate commercially prepared or self-made word and sentence lists used by the clinician to fit the needs and interests of the client. Additional topics can be generated to meet the needs and motivational level of the individual patient.

HIGH VISIBILITY

The beach is beautiful in July.
The water is blue.
Lots of people go to the beach.
People wear bathing suits for swimming at the beach.
I pack a picnic to eat at the beach.

LOW VISIBILITY

My garden is rather large.
I have a shovel and rake and a hoe.
It's very hot working in the sun.
I plant seeds for cucumbers and corn.
The vegetables are always delicious.

5. **Objective:** In a quiet therapy situation, to *comprehend* longer sentences of increasing complexity of structure (subject + verb + object + modifier/dependent clause) with the subject *not* known to the listener.

    Procedure: The listener will use visual + assistive device cues. Construct sentences that fit the listener's needs and interests. At this stage, the intent is to help the listener achieve communication competence in normal spontaneous social situations. If the listener has difficulty at the onset of this objective, have him/her relate the gist of the conversation rather than word-by-word responses. Verbatim responses are not the goal. Use repair strategies to enhance receptive skills.

    Criterion: Clinician monitoring—90% success rate.

    Materials: Any appropriate commercially prepared or self-made word and sentence lists used by the clinician to fit the needs and interests of the client. Additional topics can be generated to meet the needs and motivational level of the individual patient.

HIGH VISIBILITY

My mother and father planned the wedding all by themselves.
The bridesmaids wore blue, and the flowers were pink.
The bachelor party was on Monday night, with many friends and family there.
The wedding was beautiful and the food was wonderful.
The bride was beautiful in her mother's wedding gown.

LOW VISIBILITY

I wanted to drive my car, but I had to take the train.
I planned to start my trip in early December and left on time.
The train station was very old but recently remodeled.
I bought a ticket for $62 for a round trip to Chicago.
Sleeping on the train is an adventure that everyone should try.

C. **GOAL:** To *integrate* visual + assistive device (visual + auditory, visual + electrical, or visual + vibrotactile) inputs for the purpose of efficient receptive communication of words, phrases, and sentence-length material *without* the topic known and in the presence of low-level ambient noise. NOTE: At this point, the listener should be tested to determine the level of functioning in low-level ambient noise and then the appropriate objective chosen as a starting point. It is felt that therapy can be terminated when the listener and clinician feel that communicative competence has been attained or plateauing has occurred and no significant progress is likely to occur.

1. **Objective:** In the presence of low-level ambient noise, to *identify* target phoneme signatures from Objective 3, Goal A. Once this is achieved, sentence-length materials can be employed (see following).

2. **Objective:** In the presence of low-level ambient noise, to *comprehend* short sentences of simple structure with the subject known to the listener.
   Procedure: The listener will use visual + assistive device cues. Construct sentences that fit the listener's needs and interests. At the initiation of this objective, it is suggested that phoneme articulatory visibility and the individual acoustic/tactile signatures of the phonemes be reviewed. Use repair strategies to elicit correct responses.

   Sentences with high visibility loading will be used first, followed by sentences with low visibility loading (i.e., words with bilabial phonemes vs. lingua-alveolar phonemes).

   Low-level ambient noise can be generated by (a) radio playing, (b) static from a radio, (c) tape-recorded speech babble or cafeteria noise, or (d) recorded white noise from an audiometer. The patient should be able to detect the noise but still be able to hear the clinician's voice.

Criterion: Clinician monitoring—90% success rate.

Materials: Any appropriate commercially prepared or self-made word and sentence lists used by the clinician to fit the needs and interests of the client. Additional topics can be generated to meet the needs and motivational level of the individual patient.

HIGH VISIBILITY
The topic is presidents.

The president is elected by the people.
The president must be born in America.
John F. Kennedy was the youngest president so far.
We elect a president every 4 years.
The president lives in the White House.
There are two major political parties in America.
There has only been one bachelor president.
President Lincoln was shot at Ford Theater.
George Washington was the first man to serve in this office.
The first lady is the president's wife.

LOW VISIBILITY
The topic is going to the doctor.

You go to the doctor when you are sick.
The nurse will take your temperature.
The doctor will ask you what is wrong.
You will describe your symptoms.
The examination will take several minutes.
The doctor will look in your eyes, ears, and mouth.
He may give you a shot.
You will take your medicine three times a day.
The secretary will give you a new appointment.
Please call the doctor to say you feel fine.

3. **Objective:** In the presence of low-level ambient noise, to *comprehend* longer sentences of complex structure with the subject known to the listener.
   Procedure: Same as Objective 2, Goal C.
   Criterion: Clinician monitoring—90% success rate.
   Materials: Any appropriate commercially prepared or self-made word and sentence lists used by the clinician to fit the needs and interests of the client. Additional topics can be generated to meet the needs and motivational level of the individual patient.

HIGH VISIBILITY

The topic is family.

I live with my mother and father most of the year.
My father is 44 years old and feels fine.
My mother is 55 years old but she is very fit.
They were married in Brooklyn and lived there 20 years.
Many people were at the wedding to wish my parents well.
I have three brothers, no sisters, and a big dog named Barney.
The names of my brothers are Mathew, Bob, and Peter.
We all live in a house in Maine next to the beach.
We vacation every year in Miami during the winter months.
My brother and I go fishing on vacation all the time.

LOW VISIBILITY

The topic is tennis.

Tennis can be played on clay, grass, or asphalt.
Two people play singles but four people play doubles.
A strong serve may reach 100 miles per hour and can win the game.
It is important to concentrate so you can return the ball accurately.
Tennis is played all year long and around the world.
The big four tournaments are the Australian, French, and American Opens and Wimbledon.
The backhand is a difficult stroke to perfect and hit well.
Both men and women become professional tennis players.
The top players earn several million dollars a year.
Children may begin to learn to play tennis when they are very young.

4. **Objective:** In the presence of low-level ambient noise, to *comprehend* short sentences of simple structure with the subject *not* known to the listener.

   Procedure: Same as Objective 2, Goal C.

   Criterion: Clinician monitoring—90% success rate.

   Materials: Any appropriate commercially prepared or self-made word and sentence lists used by the clinician to fit the needs and interests of the client. Additional topics can be generated to meet the needs and motivational level of the individual patient.

HIGH VISIBILITY

Farmers grow food.
Farmers must wake up very early.
A farm has many animals.

Few families live on farms today.
Many farms are run as big businesses.
The wheat farms are very big.
Smaller farms produce milk from cows.
American farms feed many people in the world.
It is fun to live on a farm.
The farmer is a very important person.

LOW VISIBILITY

Children start kindergarten at 5 years old.
Kids enjoy kindergarten because it is fun.
After kindergarten, children go to elementary school.
Elementary school is first grade to sixth grade.
Everyone has to take gym.
Junior high school is for 3 years.
Many students study a foreign language.
High school lasts 4 years.
Not everyone goes to college.
College is usually for 4 years.

5. **Objective:** In the presence of low-level ambient noise, to *comprehend* longer sentences of complex structure with subject *not* known to the listener.

   Procedure: Same as Objective 2, Goal C.

   Criterion: Clinician monitoring—90% success rate.

   Materials: Any appropriate commercially prepared or self-made word and sentence lists used by the clinician to fit the needs and interests of the client. Additional topics can be generated to meet the needs and motivational level of the individual patient.

HIGH VISIBILITY

One of my favorite restaurants serves Mexican food.
All restaurants have a menu to list their food.
Some restaurants charge a lot of money to eat a meal.
French restaurants have fancy food and small portions.
Fast food restaurants sell food in every big city and small town.
I like to eat bacon and eggs for breakfast and drink coffee.
My friends and I go out for dinner every Friday night.
When I go on vacation, I eat all my meals at restaurants.
The best food may be found at a small family restaurant.
My family spends $40 for dinner at the Chinese restaurant.

LOW VISIBILITY

An airport is very busy during the rush hour.
The planes wait on the runway for a very long time.
Be sure to check in at the airport at least 1 hour before your flight.
When you fly, do you like to sit next to the window?
I bought my ticket from my local travel agent.
I made reservations to fly to California next week.
It costs a lot of money to park your car at the airport.
Do you check your bags or carry them on the plane yourself?
Is it important for you to sit in the nonsmoking section of the airplane?
It is nice to have someone pick you up after your flight.

6. **Objective:** In the presence of low-level ambient noise, to *comprehend* conversational speech with the subject known to the listener.
   Procedure: Spontaneous conversation regarding topics relevant to the patient, everyday events, discrimination of pictures, or card games. High and low visibility stimuli should be used.
   Criterion: Clinician monitoring—90% success rate.
   Materials: Paragraph-length material or flowing participatory conversation should be used. Sources are spontaneously generated materials reflecting the milieu of card games, adult board games, and discussion of television programs, news and sporting events, books, newspapers, and magazines.

7. **Objective:** In the presence of low-level ambient noise, to *comprehend* conversational speech with the subject *not* known to the listener.
   Procedure: Same as Objective 2, Goal C.
   Criterion: Clinician monitoring—90% sucess rate.
   Materials: Same as Objective 6, Goal C.

8. **Objective:** In the presence of higher levels of ambient noise, to *comprehend* conversational speech with the subject known to the listener. Higher level ambient noise occurs when the clinician's voice is still detectable but the noise is beginning to interfere with the input.
   Procedure: Same as Objective 2, Goal C.
   Criterion: Clinician monitoring—90% success rate.
   Materials: Same as Objective 6, Goal C.

9. **Objective:** In the presence of higher levels of ambient noise, to *comprehend* conversational speech with the subject *not* known to the listener.
   Procedure: Same as Objective 2, Goal C.
   Criterion: Clinician monitoring—90% success rate.
   Materials: Same as Objective 6, Goal C.

REFERENCES

Bhagia SU: Cochlear implant users' visual and auditory-visual performance on the Diagnostic Rhyme Test, unpublished Masters Thesis, 1992, University of California, Santa Barbara.

Binnie C, Jackson P, Montgomery A: Visual intelligibility of consonants: a lipreading screening test with implications for aural rehabilitation, *J Speech Hear Dis* 41:530-539, 1976.

Chermack GD: Information and linguistic aspects of communication. In Chermack GD: *Handbook of audiological rehabilitation*, Springfield, Ill, 1981, Charles C Thomas, pp 24-34.

Cholewiak RW, Sherrick CE: Tracking skill of a deaf person with long-term tactile aid experience: a case study, *J Rehab Res Dev* 23:20-26, 1986.

Davis H, Silverman SR: *Hearing and deafness*, New York, 1978, Holt, Rinehart & Winston, pp 536-538.

DeFilippo CL, Scott BL: A method for training and evaluating the reception of ongoing speech, *J Acoust Soc Am* 63:1186-1192, 1978.

Edgerton BJ: Rehabilitation and training of postlingually deaf adult cochlear implant patients, *Semin Hear* 6:65-90, 1985.

Fleming M: A total approach to communication therapy, *J Acad Rehab Aud* 5:28-31, 1973.

Fleming M, Birkle L, Kolman I et al: Development of workable aural rehabilitation programs, *J Acad Rehab Aud* 6:35-36, 1973.

Giolas TG: *Hearing-handicapped adults*, Englewood Cliffs, NJ, 1982, Prentice-Hall.

Green WB, Green KW: The process of speech-reading. In Northcott WH, editor: *Oral-interpreting principles and practices*, Baltimore, 1984, University Park Press.

Jackson P, Montgomery A, Binnie C: Perceptual dimensions underlying vowel lipreading performance, *J Speech Hear Res* 19:796-812, 1976.

Jeffers J, Barley M: *Look, now hear this: combined auditory training and speech reading instruction*, Springfield, Ill, 1979, Charles C Thomas.

Jeffers J, Barley M: *Speechreading (lipreading)*, Springfield, Ill, 1971, Charles C Thomas.

McCarthy P, Culpepper NB: The adult remediation process. In Alpiner JG, McCarthy PA, editors: *Rehabilitative audiology: children and adults*, Baltimore, 1987, Williams & Wilkens.

Miller G, Nicely P: An analysis of perceptual confusions among some English consonants, *J Acoust Soc Am* 27:338-352, 1955.

O'Neill JJ, Oyer H: *Visual communication for the hard of hearing*, Englewood Cliffs, NJ, 1981, Prentice-Hall.

Owens E: Consonant errors and remediation in sensorineural hearing loss, *J Speech Hear Dis* 43:331, 1978.

Owens E, Raggio M: The UCSF tracking procedure for evaluation and training of speech reception by hearing-impaired adults, *J Speech Hear Dis* 52:120-128, 1978.

Pichora-Fuller MK, Benguerel A-P: The design of CAST (computer-aided speechreading training), *J Speech Hear Res* 34:202-212, 1991.

Plant GL, Macrase JH: The NAL test development, standardization and validation, *Aust J Audiol* 4(2):62-68, 1981.

Robbins AM, Osberger MJ, Miyamoto RT et al: Speechtracking performance in single channel cochlear implant subjects, *J Speech Hear Res* 28:565-578, 1985.

Rubenstein A, Boothroyd A: Effect of two approaches to auditory training on speech recognition by hearing-impaired adults, *J Speech Hear Res* 30:153-160, 1987.

Sanders DA: *Aural rehabilitation*, Englewood Cliffs, NJ, 1982, Prentice-Hall.

Schuell H: *The Minnesota test for differential diagnosis of aphasia*, 1965, University of Minnesota Press.

Smith CR, Karp A: *A workbook in auditory training for adults*, Springfield, Ill, 1978, Charles C Thomas.

Spitzer JB, Leder SB, Milner P et al: Standardization of four videotaped tests of speechreading ranging in task difficulty, *Ear Hear* 8:227-231, 1987.

Tye-Murray N: Repair strategy usage by hearing-impaired adults and changes following communication therapy, *J Speech Rear Res* 34:921-928, 1991.

Tye-Murray N, Tyler RS: A critique of continuous discourse tracking as a test procedure, *J Speech Hear Dis* 53:226-231, 1988.

Tyler RS, Preece JP, Lowder MW: *The Iowa Cochlear Implant Tests*, Iowa City, 1983, University of Iowa.

Voiers WD: Diagnostic evaluation of speech intelligibility. In Hawley ME, editor: *Benchmark papers in acoustics*, Stroudsburg, Penn, 1977, Dowden, Hutchinson, & Roth, pp 374-387.

NAL/WEST HAVEN TEST*
Instructions

You will see a speaker saying 50 questions broken down into five categories. A written cue on the screen will inform you of each category. Please write down the *answer* to the question. Do not leave any blanks. Guess if you are not sure.

Questions About You

1. What's your last name?

2. What are your first names?

3. How old are you?

4. What's your date of birth?

5. Where were you born?

6. Are you married or single?

7. When were you married?

8. What's your job?

9. How much do you weigh?

10. How tall are you?

11. What's the color of your eyes?

12. What's your doctor's name?

*Spitzer JB, Leder SB, Milner P et al: *Ear Hear* 8:227-231, 1987.

Questions About Your Relatives

13. What is your father's name?

14. What was your mother's maiden name?

15. How many brothers do you have?

16. How many sisters do you have?

17. How many children do you have?

Questions About Your Home

18. Which town do you live in?

19. What's the name of your street?

20. Do you live in a house or an apartment?

21. What's the number of your house?

22. What's your telephone number?

23. How many bedrooms does your house have?

24. Do you have a gas or electric stove?

25. Where do you go shopping?

26. How do you get to the shops?

27. Do you have milk delivered?

Questions About Things You Like

28. What's your favorite color?

29. Do you prefer tea or coffee?

30. Which TV program do you like best?

31. Who's your favorite author?

32. Do you prefer butter or margarine?

33. What sort of pet do you like?

34. What's your favorite hobby?

Some Questions With Easy Answers

35. What's the time?

36. What day is it?

37. What color are your shoes?

38. What month comes after August?

39. What color is coal?

40. What month is it now?

41. What is 4 + 6?

42. What number comes before 26?

43. Is Peter a boy's name or a girl's name?

44. What is half of 6?

45. What day comes before Friday?

46. What language is spoken in France?

47. Is Jane a boy's name or a girl's name?

48. What is 5 + 3?

49. What color is milk?

50. What is the opposite of happy?

IOWA-KEASTER TEST—FORMS A AND B*
Instructions

You will see a speaker saying a total of 60 sentences. Please write down on your answer sheet the *sentence* you see spoken. Do not leave any blanks. Guess if you are not sure.

Form A

1. How are you?

2. Do you have a piece of paper?

3. What hours do you work?

4. Do you have a pencil?

5. Do you like to go to the movies?

6. How far is it to the post office?

7. How much time have you?

8. How far is it from here to Chicago?

9. Where do you work?

10. Did you enjoy the baseball game?

11. The train leaves at 5 o'clock.

12. Do you have an umbrella?

13. What is your favorite television program?

14. This is a cold day.

15. Have you any children?

---

*Jeffers J, Barley M: *Speechreading (lipreading)*, Springfield, Ill, 1971, Charles C Thomas.

16. How much snow did we have last night?

17. Did you finish high school?

18. Do you have chains on your car?

19. Have you ever lived in the West?

20. I'm going south for my vacation.

21. How many miles did you drive your Ford?

22. Did you get my letter?

23. What does the paper say about the weather?

24. I think it is going to snow.

25. The bank closes at 2:30 PM.

26. The snow is 5 inches deep.

27. Isn't this a beautiful day?

28. It was a perfect day for a football game.

29. You had a long distance call while you were gone.

30. It rained most of the night.

Form B

1. What time is it?

2. Do you have a dog?

3. What time did you have breakfast this morning?

4. Do you have a new car?

5. What kind of a dog do you have?

6. Have you read the newspaper this morning?

7. Where is your home?

8. How is your family?

9. Are you going home for vacation?

10. Do you like to shop?

11. Do you think it will rain this afternoon?

12. Would you like to go to the show with us?

13. What is your occupation?

14. Do you like to watch television?

15. What are your hobbies?

16. What kind of a car do you drive?

17. What day of the week is this?

18. Do you drink your coffee black?

19. My watch is slow.

20. Have you any brothers or sisters?

21. The wind is blowing from the northeast.

22. My watch doesn't keep good time.

23. What shall we do tonight?

24. Did you drive or come by train?

25. Can you have lunch with me on Friday?

26. I have an appointment at 3 o'clock.

27. Are your parents living?

28. I'll meet you at 3 o'clock.

29. You could drop me a postcard to let me know.

30. Do they allow children in that building?

CID EVERYDAY SENTENCES*
Instructions

You will be presented with 10 lists of 10 sentences (Groups A through J). Please write down on your answer sheet the *sentence* you see spoken. Do not leave any blanks. Guess if you are not sure.

List A

1. Walking's my favorite exercise.
2. Here's a nice quiet place to rest.
3. Our janitor sweeps the floors every night.
4. It would be much easier if everyone would help.
5. Good morning.
6. Open your window before you go to bed.
7. Do you think that she should stay out so late?
8. How do you feel about changing the item when we begin work?
9. Here we go.
10. Move out of the way!

List B

1. The water's too cold for swimming.
2. Why should I get up so early in the morning?
3. Here are your shoes.

---

*Davis H, Silverman SR: *Hearing and deafness*, New York, 1978, Holt, Rinehart & Winston.

4. It's raining.

5. Where are you going?

6. Come here when I call you!

7. Don't try to get out of it this time!

8. Should we let little children go the movies by themselves?

9. There isn't enough paint to finish the room.

10. Do you want an egg for breakfast?

List C

1. Everybody should brush his teeth after meals.

2. Everything's all right.

3. Don't use up all the paper when you write your letter.

4. That's right.

5. People ought to see a doctor once a year.

6. Those windows are so dirty I can't see anything outside.

7. Pass the bread and butter please!

8. Don't forget to pay your bill before the first of the month.

9. Don't let the dog out of the house.

10. There's a good ballgame this afternoon.

List D

1. It's time to go.

2. If you don't want those old magazines throw them out.

3. Do you want to wash up?

4. It's a real dark night so watch your driving.

5. I'll carry the package for you.

6. Did you forget to shut off the water?

7. Fishing in a mountain stream is my idea of a good time.

8. Fathers spend more time with their children than they used to.

9. Be careful not to break your glasses.

10. I'm sorry.

List E

1. You can catch the bus across the street.

2. Call her on the phone and tell her the news.

3. I'll catch up with you later.

4. I'll think it over.

5. I don't want to go to the movies tonight.

6. If your tooth hurts that much you ought to see a dentist.

7. Put that cookie back in the box!

8. Stop fooling around!

9. Time's up.

10. How do you spell your name?

List F

1. Music always cheers me up.

2. My brother's in town for a short while on business.

3. We live a few miles from the main road.

4. This suit needs to go to the cleaners.

5. They ate enough green apples to make them sick for a week.

6. Where have you been all this time?

7. Have you been working hard lately?

8. There's not enough room in the kitchen for a new table.

9. Where is he?

10. Look out!

List G

1. I'll see you right after lunch.

2. See you later.

3. White shoes are awful to keep clean.

4. Stand there and don't move until I tell you!

5. There's a big piece of cake left over from dinner.

6. Wait for me at the corner in front of the drugstore.

7. It's no trouble at all.

8. Hurry up!

9. The morning paper didn't say anything about rain this afternoon or tonight.

10. The phone call's for you.

List H

1. Believe me!

2. Let's get a cup of coffee.

3. Let's get out of here before it's too late.

4. I hate driving at night.

5. There was water in the cellar after that heavy rain yesterday.

6. She'll only be gone a few minutes.

7. How do you know?

8. Children like candy.

9. If we don't get rain soon, we'll have no grass.

10. They're not listed in the new phone book.

List I

1. Where can I find a place to park?

2. I like those big red apples we always get in the fall.

3. You'll get fat eating candy.

4. The show's over.

5. Why don't they paint their walls some other color.

6. What's new?

7. What are you hiding under your coat?

8. How come I should always be the one to go first?

9. I'll take sugar and cream in my coffee.

10. Wait just a minute.

List J

1. Breakfast is ready.

2. I don't know what's wrong with the car, but it won't start.

3. It sure takes a sharp knife to cut this meat.

4. I haven't read a newspaper since we bought a television set.

5. Weeds are spoiling the yard.

6. Call me a little later!

7. Do you have change for a five dollar bill?

8. How are you?

9. I'd like some ice cream with my pie.

10. I don't think I'll have any dessert.

THE GOLD RUSH PARAGRAPH*
Instructions

You will see a speaker saying a paragraph. Please watch carefully and try to understand what is said. There are six questions printed on your answer sheet. *Answer* each one to the best of your ability.

Gold was first discovered in California by a millwright named James Marshall. Marshall was building a sawmill on the banks of the American River. One morning in January 1848, as he was walking along the millrace, he saw some bright flakes at the bottom of a ditch. Marshall picked up a handful and took them back to the fort to show his partner, John Sutter. They turned out to be pure gold. Marshall and Sutter tried to keep the discovery a secret until the mill was finished, but the news spread like wildfire. Every morning gold seekers, armed with picks and shovels, came out to the sawmill. Some of them even wanted to tear the sawmill down. Marshall sent them off in all directions, telling them better places to look for gold. To his surprise they found gold everywhere. Marshall soon gained such a reputation that people would dig wherever he told them to. No one had any idea that the whole countryside was one great bed of gold.

Questions

1. In this story, did Marshall discover gold on the Rio Grande?

2. Did Marshall and Sutter try to spread the news of the discovery?

3. Did many prospectors come to the sawmill?

4. Did they tear down the sawmill?

5. Did Marshall know where the hidden deposits were?

6. Were the prospectors lucky in finding gold?

---

*Schuell H: *The Minnesota test for differential diagnosis of aphasia,* Minneapolis, 1965, University of Minnesota Press.

HELPFUL HINTS FOR THE HEARING-IMPAIRED INDIVIDUAL AND FAMILY

1. Try to face the person who is speaking to you as much as possible. Watch the person's lips, facial expressions, gestures, and body language.
2. Try to seat yourself within 6 feet of a speaker when in a friendly situation. Attempt to sit within the first several rows of seats when you are at a meeting or attending religious services. This will help you see the speaker's face and lips in order to get better input from both your assistive device and vision.
3. Ask the person to sit so that his/her face is not in shadow. Light should fall on the speaker's face and should not come from a window or other light source behind the speaker's head.
4. Try to figure out the topic that is being discussed. Your family can help by letting you know the key words being used.
5. Learn to look for the ideas being discussed. Do not get stuck on understanding every word that is being said. Use all the information you can from the environment and the speaker to get the gist of what is being said.
6. Do not be afraid to guess. If you are not sure of words, you can ask questions to try to clarify the meaning of the parts you missed.
7. You and your family should understand that it is very difficult to lipread someone whose mouth is full of food or chewing gum. Besides being rude, it interferes with the normal movements of the mouth for speech.
8. Try to relax. If you allow yourself to get tense, you will miss information and make more mistakes.
9. Try to control your own voice. This is very difficult with some forms of hearing loss, but you must try to be aware of the effort you are putting into speaking and the effect your voice has on other people. Sometimes, you can see by other people's reactions that your voice is having a negative effect. You may also ask your family to subtly let you know when you are speaking too loudly in public.
10. Try to avoid background noise whenever possible. Do not have very important information communicated to you in uncontrollably loud situations. Wait until you have left the noisy area to have the conversation.

11. Do not try to have a conversation at home when there is competition in the background. Turn off or turn down the volume of the radio or television before having a discussion. Turn off the water for the dishes or any noisy machines that interfere with hearing.

12. Do not suffer in silence. If these helpful hints are really applied and do not make a difference, you need to seek more formal assistance from an audiologist or speech-language pathologist.

CHAPTER 5

Voice and Resonance: Methods and Samples

NORMAL speech acquisition requires a combination of interrelated sensory feedback channels: visual, tactile, kinesthetic, and, most important, auditory. Once speech movement patterns are learned, they are executed within certain ranges of variability. When the normal range of variability is exceeded (i.e., a perceptible error is made), the sensory feedback channels recalibrate the production system to prevent the error from recurring (Zimmermann and Rettaliata, 1981). However, the late-deafened speaker has lost the critical auditory feedback channel and resultant information to make the necessary adjustments. The profoundly hearing-impaired or deaf speaker is unable to detect or correct the error. Over time, lack of auditory feedback causes speech degeneration (Zimmermann and Rettaliata, 1981; Binnie, Daniloff, and Buckingham, 1982; Cowie, Douglas-Cowie, and Kerr, 1982). However, the exact nature of the degeneration in the speech of the late-deafened is not currently understood.

PERCEPTUAL JUDGMENTS AND THE ADVENTITIOUSLY DEAF

Conflicting results have been reported regarding listeners' perceptual judgments and speech production abilities in the post-lingually or late-deafened adult population (Leder and Spitzer, 1990a). The controversy focuses on three main issues: (1) effects of auditory deprivation on speech and voice production; (2) criteria for determining these effects, that is, segmental (articulatory) and/or suprasegmental (prosodic) speech deterioration; and (3) appropriateness of rehabilitative intervention. The latter conflicting results are primarily a function of sample size (Cowie et al., 1982; Kirk and Edgerton, 1983; Tye, Zimmermann, and Kelso, 1983), sample criteria (Cowie, Douglas-Cowie, and Stewart, 1986; Goehl and Kaufman, 1984; Zimmermann and Collins, 1985) and use of case studies (Binnie et al., 1982; Plant, 1984; Zimmermann and Retalliata, 1981).

Pure-tone and speech discrimination abilities of the adventitiously deaf are routinely performed. In the prelingually deaf, once the hearing loss has been determined, significant effort has been directed toward analyzing the segmental errors in speech (Hudgins and Numbers; 1942, Smith, 1975). Less research, however, has been directed toward segmental and suprasegmental errors and perceptual judgments of the speech and voice of the late-deafened adult.

Some researchers, using listener judgments, have suggested that late-onset deafness does not lead to problems of speech degeneration (Espir and Rose, 1976; Goehl and Kaufman, 1984; Ling, 1976). Other studies, also using listener judgments, however, report that long-term auditory deprivation in the adventitiously deaf results in a flat, unmodulated, and dysprosodic voice with segmental speech deterioration (Penn, 1955; Kirchner and Suzuki, 1968; Elman, 1981; Ramsden, 1981; Binnie et al., 1982; Cowie et al., 1982). Such studies report that the speech of the adventitiously deaf degenerates systematically over time, indicating that auditory information plays an important role in the maintenance of normal speech.

Zimmermann and Rettaliata (1981) investigated in great detail the systematic longitudinal degeneration of speech. They concluded that the speech of the adventitiously deaf degenerated slowly due to overlearned motor patterns, errors made without knowledge of the errors occurring, and voice production changes occurring only after many instances of exceeding the normal range of variability. Articulatory movement patterns were less efficiently maintained over time when only nonauditory sensory systems were available. Therefore auditory information seems not to be used for moment-to-moment monitoring but periodically to update and calibrate the system.

Leder and Spitzer (1990a) found that acquired profound hearing loss, regardless of hearing aid use or duration of deafness, resulted in *perceptually* significant segmental and suprasegmental speech and voice quality deterioration. Subjects were 25 adventitiously deaf and 10 normal-hearing adult male speakers. Twelve subjects were classified as aidable profound and 13 subjects were classified as unaidable profound. Listeners' perceptual evaluations revealed that the aidable and unaidable adventitiously deaf subjects were judged significantly different from each other and from normal hearing subjects on all seven variables under study. The variables were, in the hierarchy of most to least disordered, intonation, pitch, rate, nasality, vowel duration, articulation, and intensity. It was concluded that auditory information is a necessary component for maintaining accurate speech and voice production abilities following onset of profound hearing loss after the acquisition of an adult phonologic system.

SPEECH ACOUSTICS AND THE ADVENTITIOUSLY DEAF

Few investigators have dealt with speech acoustics in adventitiously deaf co-chlear implant participants. In these studies, involving single participants and multiple case designs, the 3M-House single-channel cochlear implant was used (Danley and Fretz, 1982). In the study by Kirk and Edgerton (1983) on voice parameters in patients receiving cochlear implants, no precochlear implant baseline data were collected. Nonetheless, they noted that the two male subjects had voice production with lower fundamental frequency (Fo) and reduced intensity variability in the implant-on condition, in definite contrast to the implant-off condition. Conversely, their two female participants produced higher Fo voices in the implant-on condition. In both the implant-on and implant-off conditions, all four subjects produced sentences and pauses of longer duration than did normal-hearing speakers. Our case study, involving a male subject (Leder et al., 1986), used both precochlear implant and postimplant stimulation data. It was shown that the use of a single-channel cochlear implant significantly lowered Fo after the first day of stimulation. These findings also showed that reacquisition of the English contrastive stress features of Fo, intensity, and duration required an additional 4 months of cochlear implant use.

Speaking Fundamental Frequency (Fo)

Research on speaking Fo over the past 50 years has been concerned mainly with the normal developmental aspects of male (Curry, 1940; Fairbanks, Wiley, and Lassman, 1949; Mysak, 1959; Hollien and Shipp, 1972) and female (Fairbanks, Herbert, and Hammond, 1949; McGlone and Hollien, 1963; Michel, Hollein, and Moore, 1966; Stoicheff, 1981) voices. Studies of the Fo characteristics of deaf speakers have centered on the congenitally impaired and have found that individual Fo is less varied and that group Fo is higher and spans a wider range than normal (Angelocci, Kopp, and Holbrook, 1964; Boone, 1966; Nickerson, 1975; Gilbert and Campbell, 1980). Results of vowel Fo measures from a postlingually deaf adolescent indicated pubertal pitch lowering approaching normal adult Fo values (Plant, 1984). Only one study (Kirk and Edgerton, 1983) reported speaking Fo values on late-deafened men (N = 2), and it found Fo to be 30 Hz to 53 Hz higher than in their normal-hearing male subjects.

The lack of data on speaking Fo after onset of deafness in previously hearing adults limits our knowledge regarding voice quality changes in the absence of auditory feedback and thus prevents appropriate rehabilitative measures from being implemented.

In an effort to clarify these issues, Fo was investigated in a group of adventitiously profoundly hearing-impaired men (N = 21) (Leder, Spitzer, and Kirchner, 1987a) and women (N = 12) (Leder and Spitzer, 1993). Results indicated that speaking Fo was significantly higher than for normal-hearing men and women. These findings were similar to those in the literature on prelingual deafness (Angelocci et al., 1964; Boone, 1966; Nickerson, 1975; Gilbert and Campbell, 1980). It appeared that even after normal voice quality had been acquired, late-onset deafness altered speaking Fo in a direction similar to that in individuals who had never heard their own voices.

Voice Intensity

Hearing loss affects the manner in which voice intensity varies in the speech of the deaf. Sensorineural loss may cause an abnormally loud voice because of the absence of feedback via bone conduction. In contrast, conductive loss may cause a very soft voice because bone conduction allows self-monitoring of voice, which may appear very loud in comparison to the speech of other people (Miller, 1968).

Reports of intensity problems have mainly been concerned with the speech of the prelingually profoundly deaf. In such subjects, it was found that intensity problems take several forms (i.e., the voice may be too loud, too soft, or vary erratically [Miller, 1968; Martony, 1968]). We have found only one study that *quantified* intensity variations in speech of the prelingually deaf (Hood and Dixon, 1969). The authors reported that there were significant differences between deaf and normal-hearing speakers in variation of peak intensity of syllables. Specifically, deaf speakers varied intensity one half to one third less than a normal group. However, the prelingually deaf were similar to normal-hearing speakers in *pattern* of intensity changes (i.e., the deaf increased or decreased their intensity on the same syllables as normal-hearing speakers but not to the same degree).

There is a paucity of data on voice intensity changes in late-deafened adults. In the earlier reported study by Kirk and Edgerton (1983), voice intensity of two male and two female cochlear implant subjects was measured. The range of relative intensity was not significantly different between the deaf and normal-hearing subjects or in the deaf group when the cochlear implant was on or off.

Voice intensity values were also investigated in the speech of a group (N = 19) of adventitiously deaf male speakers (Leder et al., 1987b) and in a group (N = 12) of adventitiously deaf female speakers (Leder and Spitzer, 1993). Results indicated that voice intensity of oral reading was significantly increased for late-deafened adult males and females compared to normal-hearing male and female speakers. Standard deviations for deaf speakers were more than two and three times greater than normal-hearing speakers, which indicated that deaf speakers produced greater intensity fluctuations during speech. The broad fluctuations in intensity, as measured during oral reading and observed in conversational speech, contradict anecdotal reports of flat, unmodulated, and monotonous vocal quality in the speech of the adventitiously deaf (Silverman and Calvert, 1978; Ramsden,

1981). Therefore we conclude that adventitious profound deafness and resultant lack of adequate auditory feedback are associated with a significantly increased voice intensity level and greater fluctuations in intensity production. When adequate feedback was provided, intensity was reduced and, over time, approximated values of normal-hearing speakers, as indicated in a cochlear implant case study (Leder et al., 1986).

Speaking Rate

It is well documented that the prelingually deaf speak at a much slower rate than normal-hearing persons (Voelker, 1935, 1938; John and Howarth, 1965; Boone, 1966; Hood and Dixon, 1969; Nickerson et al., 1974; Nickerson, 1975). Specifically, prelingually deaf children speak at one fourth the rate of normal-hearing children and adults (Voelker, 1935), and, even after practice, the deaf children's utterance rate is less than half that of normal-hearing children and adults (Voelker, 1938). In a more recent study (John and Howarth, 1965), it was shown that duration of monosyllabic words spoken in conversational speech by prelingually deaf children was nearly double that for the same words produced by normal-hearing children. Also, when oral reading was used, sentence duration for prelingually deaf adult speakers was found to be 2 to 3.5 times greater than for normal-hearing adults (Hood and Dixon, 1969).

In addition to the gross speaking rate differences noted, studies that investigated the finer aspects of speech timing in the prelingually deaf population found many fine timing errors. For example, prolongation of speech segments (Hudgins and Numbers, 1942; Levitt, Smith, and Stromberg, 1976; Parkhurst and Levitt, 1978), insertion of long pauses at syntactically inappropriate junctures (Nickerson et al., 1974; Stark and Levitt, 1974; Osberger and Levitt, 1979), maintenance of segment durations despite changes in phonetic environment (Monsen, 1974), and an inability to differentiate temporally stressed vs. unstressed syllables (Nickerson et al., 1974) have been reported.

Speaking rate was found to be significantly correlated with intelligibility of speech and was at least as important as articulation for speech intelligibility in the prelingually deaf (Hudgins and Numbers, 1942). It has been reported that profound adventitious deafness in adults (Cowie et al., 1982; McGarr and Harris, 1983; Kirk and Edgerton, 1983), adolescents (Plant, 1984), and children (Binnie et al., 1982) resulted in speech timing errors and articulation deterioration. All but one (Cowie et al., 1982) of these investigations were single-subject designs.

There have been only a handful of studies dealing with durational aspects of speech in late-deafened adults. In case reports, Kirk and Edgerton (1983) found that hearing-impaired speakers produced sentences and pauses of longer duration than normal-hearing speakers, and Leder et al. (1986) reported a similar finding for words and syllables.

Only two studies have investigated durational aspects with group data. The first, (Leder et al., 1987c) reported group (N = 25) data on speaking rate and speaking duration on the speech of adventitiously profoundly hearing-impaired adult males, and the second dealt with the same topic and used group (N = 12) data with adventitiously profoundly hearing-impaired adult females (Leder and Spitzer, 1993.) The results indicated that speaking rate (i.e., syllables per second) was significantly slower and speaking duration was correspondingly significantly longer for late-deafened adult males and females than for normal-hearing control subjects. The significantly slower speaking rate of the late-deafened group did not cause their speech to be unintelligible but did affect overall quality. If speech becomes too labored and tedious, it may lead to reduction in use or, in severe cases, rejection of speech (John and Howarth, 1965). Therefore the 35% increase in duration for the total paragraph observed in Leder et al. (1987c) and the 27% increase in total paragraph duration observed in Leder and Spitzer (1993) may negatively affect overall speech communication.

CASE STUDY 5.1

R.S. was a 61-year-old male with bilateral complete sensorineural deafness. No response was obtained at any frequency up to the maximum output of the audiometer (Grason-Stadler, model GSI10). No hearing aid was ever worn nor was he aidable. R.S. had normal hearing until the age of 19, when he lost his hearing after contracting meningitis.

He was an articulate man who held a responsible position at a university. R.S.'s voice quality was characterized by inappropriately high pitch and fluctuating intensity control, as determined by two experienced clinicians. No gross articulation errors were noted.

Precochlear implant, R.S. was unable to produce the acoustic correlates of contrastive stress correctly (i.e., Fo, duration, and intensity). A 3M-House cochlear implant was used to provide electrical stimulation to the auditory nerve. Hearing 1 day after stimulation resulted in significantly higher Fo for initial and final stressed vs. unstressed syllables. Four months poststimulation, R.S. maintained significantly higher Fo on stressed syllables, as well as generalization of significantly increased intensity and longer syllable duration differences for all stressed vs. unstressed syllables. Perceptually, listeners judged R.S.'s contrastive stress placement as incorrect precochlear implant and as always correct postcochlear implant.

R.S.'s contrastive stress production was perceived as correct 1 day after stimulation and before any aural rehabilitation because R.S. altered Fo for stressed vs. unstressed syllables. Aural rehabilitation provided after stimulation may have contributed to reacquisition of duration and intensity cues although no direct rehabilitation focused on contrastive stress. Our program's training and continued use of the implant may have enhanced R.S.'s ability to reacquire Fo, duration, and intensity cues made available through electrical stimulation.

SUMMARY

The quantitative group acoustic data on adult male and female voice characteristics secondary to late-onset deafness are clear cut. Specifically, there is increased Fo (Leder et al., 1987a; Leder and Spitzer, 1993), greater intensity (Leder et al., 1987b; Leder and Spitzer, 1993), and longer speaking duration (i.e., a slower speaking rate [Leder et al., 1987c; Leder and Spitzer, 1993] during oral reading for late-deafened adult subjects when compared with normal-hearing controls.

REHABILITATION

The goal of voice rehabilitation is to train the hearing aid user, cochlear implantee, or vibrotactile wearer to identify and relate the enhanced auditory, electrical, or tactile information provided by the device to auditory patterns known before profound deafness and then to use the learned patterns for long-term self-monitoring (Abberton, Fourcin, and Rosen, 1985). Leder and Spitzer (1990b) have shown that longitudinal auditory feedback alone did not significantly change speech or voice production skills. It has been shown that both speech perception and production feedback rehabilitation using auditory and visual modalities allow identification of linguistic speech production rules not readily apparent by auditory information alone (e.g., production of rising/falling pitch, signaling questions/statements, and improving voice frequency range [Abberton et al., 1985]). It appears that individuals with hearing aids, cochlear implants, or vibrotactile devices may benefit from audiovisual feedback to identify, improve, and monitor speech production skills. However, neither the specific types of acoustic cues nor their hierarchy of importance for speech production are known at this time.

Although the single-channel cochlear implant's main benefit is as an aid to speechreading (Owens and Telleen, 1981; Dowel et al., 1982), the implant does provide time and intensity cues that enable the wearer to differentiate syllable duration and number of syllables (Bilger, 1977; Berliner and Eisenberg, 1987) and stress placement (Leder et al., 1986). The multichannel cochlear implant allows for enhanced pitch, Fo perception, and second formant information (Tong et al., 1982), and, in some implantees, allows for speech perception without visual input. It has been reported (Leder and Spitzer, 1990b) that input from a single-channel implant lowered speaking Fo, reduced intensity, and shortened speaking duration; all approximating measures obtained from normal-hearing speakers. Voice rehabilitation with the goal of lowering Fo and overall pitch would be beneficial to both single- and multi-channel cochlear implant and vibrotactile users and selected hearing aid wearers.

Late-onset deaf speakers exhibited increased voice intensity while maintaining appropriate general American English breath groups and phrasing (Leder et al., 1987b). Voice rehabilitation, therefore, should focus on decreasing overall voice intensity and reducing erratic intensity fluctuations, with the knowledge that appropriate breath groups and phrase structure have been maintained.

The literature dealing with the prelingually deaf has reported that teaching the appropriate durational characteristics of speech improved speech rhythm (John and Howarth, 1965; Hood and Dixon, 1969), which enhanced speech intelligibility (Hudgins and Numbers, 1942). It would be advantageous, therefore, to stress appropriate rate of speech during voice rehabilitation with late-deafened speakers who exhibit rate abnormalities. An effective method would focus on decreasing phonation time of syllables and words, which, in turn, would increase the rate of syllables per second. Successful therapy would have to be directed toward using the intact visual, tactile, and kinesthetic sensory feedback channels because of the paucity of available auditory input.

A technique to increase speaking rate is speechtracking (DeFilippo and Scott, 1978). Speechtracking provides speech production rehabilitation as well as speech reception training. In this technique, rate of the incoming message determines rate of speech production, so a range of increasing speaking rates can be implemented. Self-monitoring of speech output is required by the subject in order to match the rate, sound, feel, and look of the incoming message. Therefore, voice rehabilitation would have the dual purpose of improving the late-deafened speaker's speech rhythm and making speech more natural sounding. Speechtracking is discussed as a method to practice speechreading in Chapter 4.

THERAPY PLANS: GOALS, OBJECTIVES, AND SUCCESS CRITERIA
General Guidelines

Any habitual use of inappropriate voice pitch, resonance, intensity, rate, or articulation in late-deafened adults should be corrected. An assistive device should always be used during therapy, and its particular input signature must be learned and self-monitored by the person. Therefore, a stimulus item should be presented with the desired pitch, resonance, intensity, rate, and correct articulation using visual input and input from the chosen assistive device (i.e., enhanced auditory, electrical, or vibrotactile).

It must be remembered that the late-deafened individual has previously acquired all of these verbal skills but now requires relearning to eliminate any deterioration that may have occurred as a result of the hearing loss. If the new enhanced auditory, electrical, or vibrotactile inputs are not paired and learned in conjunction with the appropriate verbal cues, the person cannot use the assistive device optimally. In other words, the person's stored referent for an acoustic event must be reactivated and paired correctly with the novel input from the assistive device and visual cues when appropriate.

A hierarchic therapy approach follows. Active patient participation is required because only the patient can ultimately integrate the verbal cues with the novel input from the assistive device and relate them to previously learned patterns. With the assistive device functioning, the feedback loop is once again closed for the person; therefore self-monitoring following correct relearning is essential for overall success and long-term maintenance.

Instrumentation

Visual feedback is essential for therapy with the late-deafened assistive device user. A variety of instruments can be used, many of which are readily available (e.g., VU meter of audiometer, tape recorder, audiometer, sound-level meter, commercially available voice analyzers [Kay Elemetrics Visi-Pitch]), and stop watch). The goal is to have the speaker match the appropriate visual/vocal feedback from the instrumentation, thereby learning correct vocal modulation of pitch, loudness, and stress/rhythm.

Voice: Rationale for Therapy

Late-deafened individuals are often unable to detect normal pitch and intensity used in conversational speech. The inability to monitor their own voice production produces a voice quality generally higher in both pitch and loudness than is considered to be socially acceptable. The inability to monitor these parameters also leads to loss of the prosody of speech, which normally adds meaning to communication.

Therapy protocol. The goals and objectives included in this manual are designed for individuals who are using visual feedback plus enhanced auditory, electrical, or tactile modalities. As progress is made, the visual system can be gradually phased out as the person learns to become more aware of the feedback cues provided by the assistive device.

Resonance: Rationale for Therapy

The late-deafened adult often produces speech with constant or inappropriate nasal resonance. Hyper- or hyponasal resonance often leads the listener to make a negative judgment concerning the speaker. Severely disordered nasal resonance also decreases intelligibility. It is appropriate to attempt to normalize nasal resonance in the late-deafened speaker who exhibits abnormal nasal resonance in order to improve both social acceptance and communicative skills.

Therapy protocol. Initiating therapy with a visual feedback system provides the individual with a readily identifiable starting point for monitoring nasality. It is important that the client understand that some sounds are meant to be produced with nasal resonance and to be able to identify them. Contrastive pairs help to teach how meaning is changed by the distinctive features of presence vs. absence of nasality and stop vs. continuant. Reading provides an additional cue to the presence or absence of nasality before production. A gradual transfer from reading to spontaneous speech and from clinician to client monitoring allows for the the development of awareness of enhanced auditory, electrical, or vibrotactile cues to monitor correct production.

Articulation: Rationale for Therapy

The speech-sound production of the late-deafened adult deteriorates because of lack of adequate auditory feedback. Usually, the phonemes with high frequency characteristics (i.e., /s,z,f,v,t,k,tʃ,ʃ/) deteriorate first and are distorted the most. Nonvisible phonemes also deteriorate. The changes in articulatory precision, although not resulting in gross articulation errors and significant intelligibility changes, can produce a negative social attitude toward the late-deafened speaker.

Therapy protocol. Articulation errors are identified using standard testing procedures and are grouped by spectral characteristics and speechreading visibility features. Standard articulation rehabilitation techniques are used to teach correct production of the target phonemes. It is stressed to the individual that improvement in articulation will enhance overall communicative ability, both expressively and receptively, by increasing awareness of speech-sound production and enhancing speechreading skills.

A. **GOAL:** To *produce* a pitch level appropriate for age and sex in conversational speech (for purposes of rehabilitation the term "pitch" will be substituted for frequency).

  1. **Objective:** To *understand* the concept of pitch as it relates to voice and speech production and how pitch affects listener's comprehension and judgment.
    Procedures:
    a. Didactic presentation of the concepts, including typical pitch patterns in English sentence types (e.g., declaratives, interrogatives, imperatives).
    b. Illustration of low pitch and high pitch using a visual display on a piece of equipment such as a commercially available voice/pitch analysis unit or using arm gesture paired with low vs. high stimulus comparisons. For patients with musical backgrounds, illustrations using written music or an instrument can be employed.
    c. Low vs. high stimuli may be paired with tactile feedback in which the patient feels the larynx of the instructor and compares with his/her own

larynx. This is particularly effective as an illustrative strategy if there is a large difference in Fo between the instructor and the patient or other persons who may serve as examples.

Criterion: Patient appears to understand the concept; ongoing assessment.

Materials:

a. Vocabulary: Low pitch, high pitch, rising and falling pitch, pitch associated with meanings (i.e., questions, statements, declaratives)
b. Commercially available voice/pitch analyzer
c. Musical instruments
d. Graphic illustrations of high vs. low pitch

2. **Objective:** To *practice* using low and high pitch in a non-word context.

Procedure: Using the visual feedback system, the clinician will demonstrate open vowel production using a low pitch and a high pitch. The patient will then imitate the clinician's productions. The clinician should point out the patient's accuracy using visual feedback and encourage the patient to make use of other cues (i.e., enhanced auditory, electrical, or vibrotactile with their assistive device and/or kinesthetic via the larynx).

Criterion: Clinician monitoring— 100% success rate.

Materials: All general American English vowels.

3. **Objective::** To *produce* speech at appropriate pitch with no ambient noise.

Procedure: This step requires the clinician to make a judgment regarding the patient's habitual pitch and its appropriatness. From data gathered during the assessment phase, objective information is obtained that documents how far the patient deviates from the mean for age and gender. If voice analysis equipment is available for therapy, then the assessment/baseline data may be used at this point and as a continual referent for progress. Introduce the visual feedback system and obtain a baseline reading.

Using a visual feedback instrument, if available, establish consistent use of appropriate target pitches in a single-word environment. Gradually decrease visual feedback and replace with clinician monitoring at the sentence level.

When visual feedback has been eliminated, repeat the described procedure, gradually replacing clinician monitoring with self-monitoring with the individual's assistive device until the criterion is met.

Criterion: Self-monitoring—90% success rate.

Materials: Any appropriate commercially prepared or self-made word and sentence lists used by the clinician to fit the needs and interests of the client. Additional topics can be generated to meet the needs and motivational level of the individual patient.

One-syllable words

beet	deem	feet
pick	sip	bin
bed	met	said
man	hand	land
pot	crop	shot
food	brute	loot
put	soot	but
coat	bone	goat
caught	fought	bought

Sentences

Is feeding time at the zoo 3 o'clock?

The bids for the antiques were too high for me!

Be sure to mention that your hearing aid is broken.

The band played and everyone clapped their hands.

Stop driving your car so far from home!

Her bathing suit was beautiful and unique.

Please put the book back in the bookcase!

Is a home run the goal in baseball?

The cat caught its paw in the faucet!

4. **Objective:** To *produce* speech in therapy at appropriate pitch with low background environmental noise.

   Procedure: See Objective 3, Goal A. Begin at sentence level with visual feedback. Introduce low-level background noise (tape recording or sitting outdoors in an area with low-level environmental sounds).

   Criterion: Self-monitoring—90% success rate.

   Materials: Any appropriate commercially prepared or self-made word and sentence lists used by the clinician to fit the needs and interests of the client. Additional topics can be generated to meet the needs and motivational level of the individual patient.

Sentences

Was the stream clean and cool that evening?

The fish was delicious and it was not expensive.

Putting a child to bed is never any fun!

My back has an ache that is annoying!

The model posed on the marble table?

A tube of toothpaste costs two dollars?

The soot in the chimney was a foot thick!

I hope you told them that I don't want to go!

Often, I feel awfully bad in August.

5. **Objective:** To *produce* speech in therapy at appropriate pitch with low-level conversation as background.

    Procedure: See Objective 3, Goal A. Use tape recording of conversation as background or conduct training in a cafeteria.

    Criterion: Self-monitoring—90% success rate.

    Materials: Conversational areas might include topics of interest to the patient, current events, sports, television programs, etc.

6. **Objective:** To *produce* speech at appropriate pitch in actual social situations with varying types of background noise.

    Procedure: See Objective 3, Goal A. Begin at sentence or conversational level with clinican monitoring. Gradually decrease clinician control until spontaneous situations are used.

    Criterion: Self monitoring—90% success rate.

    Materials: Conversational areas might include topics of interest to the patient, current events, sports, television programs, etc. Suggest group sessions and controlled social situations (card games) arranged by clinician.

B. **GOAL:** To *produce* a loudness level appropriate for the conversational situation. Suggested materials: any visual feedback system (sound-level meter, VU meter) and sentence-length material (for purposes of rehabilitation the term "loudness" will be substituted for intensity).

1. **Objective:** To *understand* the concept of loudness as it relates to voice and speech production and affects communication efficiency and listener judgment.

    Procedure:

    a. Didactic presentation of the concepts, including typical loudness patterns that convey emotional information (e.g., yelling in anger, whispering in confidence).

    b. Illustration of quiet vs. loud production using a visual display on a piece of equipment such as a commercially available voice/pitch analysis unit, VU meter of audiometer or tape recorder, or using arm gesture paired with quiet vs. loud vs. very loud stimulus comparisons. The concept of socially appropriate conversational loudness is introduced. The social disadvantage of inappropriate loudness is discussed.

       For patients with musical backgrounds, illustrations using written music or an instrument can be employed.

    c. Quiet vs. loud stimuli may be paired with tactile feedback in which the patient feels the larynx of the instructor and compares with his/her own larynx. This is particularly effective as an illustrative strategy if there is a large difference in loudness between the instructor and the patient or other persons who may serve as examples.

Criterion: Patient appears to understand the concept; ongoing assessment.

Materials: Any appropriate commercially prepared or self-made word and sentence lists used by the clinician to fit the needs and interests of the client. Additional topics can be generated to meet the needs and motivational level of the individual patient.

  a. Vocabulary: Quiet, loud, very loud, and loudness associated with different contexts and emotional content

  b. Commercially available voice/pitch analyzer, VU meter of audiometer, tape recorder

  c. Musical instruments

  d. Graphic illustrations of quiet vs. loud vs. very loud

2. **Objective:** To *practice* using quiet and loud intensity in a vowel environment and word context.

Procedure: Using the visual feedback system, the clinician demonstrates open vowel production using quiet, loud, and very loud productions. The patient then imitates the clinician's productions. The clinician should point out the patient's accuracy using visual feedback and encourage the patient to make use of other cues (i.e., as enhanced audiory, electrical, or vibrotactile with the assistive device and/or kinesthetic via the larynx). Repeat with sentence-length material.

Criterion: Clinician monitoring— 100% success rate.

Materials: Any appropriate commercially prepared or self-made word and sentence lists used by the clinician to fit the needs and interests of the client. Additional topics can be generated to meet the needs and motivational level of the individual patient.

Vowels

All general American English vowels.

Sentences

My feet hurt even when I wear sneakers.
The middle-man sells pickles in the city.
She met her husband Ned on Wednesday?
The landing craft was designed for Mars.
The pot was so hot that Harriet dropped it!
Riding boots should be worn to protect the feet.
The root system of the rhododendron is very superficial.
Sonya wrote a whole book about boating?
They sought a solution to the problem.

3. **Objective:** To *produce* speech at appropriate loudness with no ambient noise.

   Procedure: This objective requires the clinician to make a judgment regarding the patient's habitual loudness level and its appropriateness. From data gathered during the assessment phase, objective information is obtained that documents how far the patient deviates from normal loudness levels (i.e., approximately 40 to 50 dB HL in conversational speech). If voice analysis equipment is available for therapy, then assessment/baseline data may be used as this point and as a continual referent for progress. Introduce the visual feedback system and obtain a baseline reading.

   Criterion: Self-monitoring—90% success rate.

   Materials: Any appropriate commercially prepared or self-made word and sentence lists used by the clinician to fit the needs and interests of the client. Additional topics can be generated to meet the needs and motivational level of the individual patient.

   Sentences

   Our school's team won at the swim meet.
   I wish you'd stop picking on me!
   Carmen said she'd head for the Netherlands?
   That man has excellent eye-hand coordination.
   Will you stop playing that rotten song?
   His rudeness interferred with the group's progress!
   Please cut down the heat pump's noise!
   He caught his toe on the garden hose.
   The horse was loose on *our* lawn?

4. **Objective:** To *produce* speech with appropriate loudness in therapy with low background environmental noise.

   Procedure: See Objective 3, Goal B. Begin at the sentence level. Introduce low-level background noise (tape recording or sitting outdoors in an area with low-level environmental sounds).

   Criterion: Self-monitoring—90% success rate.

   Materials: Any appropriate commercially prepared or self-made word and sentence lists used by the clinician to fit the needs and interests of the client. Additional topics can be generated to meet the needs and motivational level of the individual patient.

   Sentences

   He committed treason in the Eastern Congo.
   Atlantic City is a pretty city in summer.

It was getting rather late for picking red berries.
The actress ran across the stage and fainted.
Was the parson angry about the carpet?
Was Howard fooled by her aloof behavior?
Does Mr. Jones like tomatoes in his salad?
The flaw in the porch became obvious in Autumn.

5. **Objective:** To *produce* speech with appropriate loudness in therapy with low-level conversation as background.

   Procedure: See Objective 3, Goal B. Use tape recording of conversation as background or conduct training in a cafeteria.

   Criterion: Self-monitoring—90% success rate.

   Materials: Any appropriate commercially prepared or self-made word and sentence lists used by the clinician to fit the needs and interests of the client. Additional topics can be generated to meet the needs and motivational level of the individual patient.

Sentences

Was your dream about the birds and the bees?
The House of Peers helps rule England.
Did Mary grow the best pear in the fair?
Are penguins found in Antartica?
The shop closed early!
The wolf looked over the rough barnyard.
The Aswan Dam chokes the normal flow of the Nile.
Did you arrive in Boston before four in the morning?

6. **Objective:** To *produce* speech with appropriate loudness in actual social situations with varying types of background noise.

   Procedure: Begin at conversational level with clinician monitoring. Suggest group sessions, controlled social situations (card games) arranged by clinician. Gradually decrease clinician control until spontaneous situations are used.

   Criterion: Self monitoring—90% success rate.

   Materials: Conversational areas might include topics of interest to the patient, current events, sports, television programs, etc. Suggest group sessions and controlled social situations (card games) arranged by clinician.

Sentences

The player in Trinidad beat the steel drum.
She still forgets to take her heart pills!
Did Henry's headache force him to bed?
The manager was happy to see our large party.

I'm sorry I borrowed your watch without asking!
Irish stew is her favorite food.
The butcher brushed the counter clear and put the duck on it.
She lives a stone's throw from London!
The knights fought the war riding on large draft horses.

C. GOAL: To *use* pitch and loudness modulation to *produce* normal prosody during conversation in varying situations. Suggested materials are the same as in Goals A and B.

1. **Objective:** To *understand* how pitch and loudness variations are used in normal conversation and detected by the assistive device used by the individual.
   Procedure: Same as in Goals A and B.
   Criterion: Open discussion, ongoing.
   Materials: Same as in Goals A and B.

2. **Objective:** To *produce* appropriate pitch and loudness modulation during therapy in role-playing situations with no background noise.
   Procedure: Use structured situations (e.g., clinician questions and patient responds and vice versa).
   Criterion: Self-monitoring—90% success rate.
   Materials: Same as in Goals A and B.

3. **Objective:** To *produce* appropriate pitch and loudness modulation during therapy in role-playing situations with low-level background noise (environmental, conversation, and combination).
   Procedure: See Objective 2, Goal C. Introduce tape-recorded or natural background noise. Begin with clinician monitoring and gradually replace with self-monitoring.
   Criterion: Self-monitoring—90% success rate.
   Materials: Same as in Goals A and B.

4. **Objective:** To *produce* appropriate frequency and loudness modulation in actual social situations with varying types and intensities of background noise.
   Procedure: Begin with clinician monitoring and gradually replace with self-monitoring.
   Criterion: Self-monitoring—90% success rate.
   Materials: Same as in Goals A and B.

D. GOAL: To *produce* conversational speech with appropriate oral and nasal resonance. Suggested materials are mirrors, nasal flow indicator, nasal/non-nasal word pairs.

1. **Objective:** To *understand* how oral vs. nasal resonance is used to distinguish speech sounds and to identify /m, n, ŋ/ as being produced with nasal resonance.

   Procedure: Didactic presentation of the concept of nasal resonance. Illustration of oral vs. nasal resonance using the three English nasal phonemes and the patient's assistive device. Patient is to identify non-nasal vs. nasal phonemes.

   Criterion: Patient appears to understand the concept; 100% correct identification; ongoing assessment.

   Materials: General American English vowels and non-nasal consonants paired with prolongations of /m, n, ŋ/.

2. **Objective:** To *produce* oral/nasal word pairs as directed by the clinician.

   Procedure: Have person read or name pictures of oral/nasal word pairs. Gradually transfer from clinician monitoring to self-monitoring.

   Criterion: Self-monitoring—90% success rate.

   Materials:

   WORD PAIRS

Nasal		*Non-Nasal*	
man	nanny	tap	batter
mean	nimble	beet	fever
moan	neon	coat	boulder
mine	normal	type	fortress
moon	nine	soup	tissue
money	ring	table	sip
many	song	wallet	bought
mommy	hang	building	had
mini	cling	baby	click
manly	bang	whisper	bat
none	singing	suck	sitting
nine	beaming	kick	beating
noon	charming	toot	charting
name	tanning	cake	talking
Nan	winning	ace	wishing

3. **Objective:** To *produce* oral and nasal sounds appropriately in sentences while reading.

   Procedure: Begin reading with clinician monitoring and gradually transfer to self-monitoring.

   Criterion: Self-monitoring—90% success rate.

Materials: Use newspaper and magazine articles. Underline the nasal phonemes so the patient can be cued to concentrate on correct production.

4. **Objective:** To *produce* oral and nasal sounds appropriately in sentences spoken spontaneously and in conversational speech.

Procedure: Present pictures or other appropriate stimuli and ask the person to produce sentences in conversational speech. Begin with structured conversation in the therapy setting. Gradually expand to natural settings and social situations. Transfer from clinician monitoring to self-monitoring.

Criterion: Self-monitoring—90% success rate.

Materials: Pictures or objects, current events, group discussions on topics of interest.

E. **GOAL:** To *produce* conversational speech with appropriate phrasing and breath groups.

1. **Objective:** To *understand* how phrasing and breath groups are used to produce speech with normal rhythm and flow.

Procedure: Didactic presentation of the concepts of phrasing and breath groups and the ability to produce speech with normal rhythm (i.e., not too many or too few words per breath). See Goal B for maintenance of normal intensity patterns during speech production.

Criterion: Patient appears to understand the concept; 100% correct identification; ongoing assessment.

Materials: Illustration of appropriate general American English phrasing and breath groups by the clinician using graphic and conversational material.

2. **Objective:** To *produce* appropriate English phrasing and breath groups.

Procedure: Have patient read from newspaper or magazine articles. Gradually transfer from clinician monitoring to self-monitoring.

Criterion: Self-monitoring—90% success rate.

Materials: Any printed material with appropriate phrase length first marked and then unmarked to allow for the patient to generalize correct use of phrase length and breath group.

3. **Objective:** To *produce* phrase length and breath groups appropriately in sentences spoken spontaneously and in conversational speech.

Procedure: Present pictures or other appropriate stimuli and ask the person to produce sentences in conversational speech. Begin with structured conversation in the therapy setting. Gradually expand to natural settings and social situations. Transfer from clinician monitoring to self-monitoring.

Criterion: Self-monitoring—90% success rate.

Materials: Pictures or objects, current events, group discussions on topics of interest.

REFERENCES

Abberton E, Fourcin AJ, Rosen S: Speech perceptual and productive rehabilitation in electro-cochlear stimulation. In Schindler RA, Merzenich MM, editors: *Cochlear implants*, New York, 1985, Raven Press, pp 527-537.

Angelocci AA, Kopp GA, Holbrook A: The vowel formants of deaf and normal hearing 11- to 14-year old boys, *J Speech Hear Dis* 29:156-170, 1964.

Berliner KI, Eisenberg LS: Our experience with cochlear implants: have we erred in our expectations? *Am J Otol* 8:222-229, 1987.

Bilger RC: Psychoacoustic evaluation of present prostheses, *Ann Otol Rhinol Laryngol* 86(suppl 38):92-140, 1977.

Binnie CA, Daniloff RG, Buckingham HW: Phonetic disintegration in a five-year-old following sudden hearing loss, *J Speech Hear Dis* 47:181-189, 1982.

Boone DR: Modification of the voices of deaf children, *Volta Rev* 68:686-694, 1966.

Cowie R, Douglas-Cowie E, Kerr AG: A study of speech deterioration in post-lingually deafened adults, *J Laryngol Otol* 96:101-112, 1982.

Cowie R, Douglas-Cowie E, Stewart P: A response to Goehl and Kaufman (1984), *J Speech Hear Dis* 51:183-187, 1986.

Curry ET: The pitch characteristics of the adolescent male voice, *Speech Monogr* 7:48-62, 1940.

Danley MJ, Fretz R: Design and functioning of the single-channel cochlear implant. In House WF, Berliner KI, editors: Cochlear implants: progress and perspectives, *Ann Otol Rhinol Laryngol* 91(Suppl 91):21-26, 1982.

DeFilippo CL, Scott BL: A method for training and evaluating the reception of ongoing speech, *J Acoust Soc Am* 63:1186-1192, 1978.

Dowel R, Martin L, Tong Y et al: A 12-consonant confusion study on a multiple-channel cochlear implant patient, *J Speech Hear Res* 25:509-516, 1982.

Elman J: Effects of frequency shifted feedback on the pitch of vocal production, *J Acoust Soc Am* 70:45-50, 1981.

Espir MLE, Rose FC: *Basic neurology of speech*, Oxford, 1976, Blackwell.

Fairbanks G, Wiley JH, Lassman FM: An acoustical study of vocal pitch in 7- and 8-year-old boys, *Child Dev* 20:63-69, 1949.

Fairbanks G, Herbert EL, Hammond JM: An acoustical study of vocal pitch in 7- and 8-year-old girls, *Child Dev* 20:71-78, 1949.

Gilbert HR, Campbell MI: Speaking fundamental frequency in three groups of hearing-impaired individuals, *J Commun Dis* 13:195-205, 1980.

Goehl H, Kaufman D: Do the effects of adventitious deafness include disordered speech? *J Speech Hear Dis* 49:58-64, 1984.

Hollien H, Shipp T: Speaking fundamental frequency and chronological age in males, *J Speech Hear Res* 15:155-159, 1972.

Hood RB, Dixon RF: Physical characteristics of speech rhythm of deaf and normal-hearing speakers, *J Comm Dis* 2:20-28, 1969.

Hudgins DV, Numbers FC: An investigation of intelligibility of speech of the deaf, *Genet Psychol Monogr* 25:289-292, 1942.

John JEJ, Howarth JN: The effect of time distortions on the intelligibility of deaf children's speech, *Lang Speech* 8:127-134, 1965.

Kirchner S, Suzuki Y: Laryngeal reflexes and voice production, *NY Acad Sci* 155:98-129, 1968.

Kirk KI, Edgerton BJ: Effects of cochlear implant use on voice parameters, *Otolaryngol Clin North Am* 16:281-292, 1983.

Leder SB, Spitzer JB: A perceptual evaluation of the speech of adventitiously deaf adult males, *Ear Hear* 11:169-175, 1990a.

Leder SB, Spitzer JB: Longitudinal effects of single-channel cochlear implantation on voice quality, *Laryngoscope* 100:395-398, 1990b.

Leder SB, Spitzer JB: Speaking fundamental frequency, intensity, and rate of adventitiously profoundly hearing-impaired adult women, *J Acoust Soc Am* 93:2146-2151, 1993.

Leder SB, Spitzer JB, Milner P et al: Vibrotactile stimulation for the adventitiously deaf: an alternative to cochlear implantation, *Arch Phys Med* 67:754-758, 1986.

Leder SB, Spitzer JB, Milner P et al: Reacquisition of contrastive stress in an adventitiously deaf speaker using a single-channel cochlear implant, *J Acoust Soc Am* 79:1967-1974, 1986.

Leder SB, Spitzer JB, Kirchner JC: Speaking fundamental frequency of postlingually profoundly deaf adult men, *Ann Otol Rhinol Laryngol* 96:322-324, 1987a.

Leder SB, Spitzer JB, Flevaris-Phillips C et al: Voice intensity of prospective cochlear implant candidates and normal hearing adult males, *Laryngoscope* 97:224-227, 1987b.

Leder SB, Spitzer JB, Kirchner JC, et al: Speaking rate of adventitioulty deaf male cochlear implant candidates, *J Acoust Soc Am* 82:843-846, 1987c.

Levitt H, Smith CR, Stromberg H: Acoustical, articulatory, and perceptual characteristics of the speech of deaf children, In Fant G, editor: *Proceedings of the speech communication seminar*, New York, 1976, Wiley, pp 129-139.

Ling D: *Speech and the hearing impaired child: therapy and practice*, Washington, DC, 1976, The Alexander Graham Bell Association for the Deaf.

Martoney J: On the correction of the voice pitch level for severely hard of hearing subjects, *Am Ann Deaf* 113:195-202, 1968.

McGarr NS, Harris KS: Articulatory control in a deaf speaker. In Hochberg, Levitt H, Osberger MJ, editors: *Speech of the hearing impaired: research, training, and personnel preparation*, Baltimore, 1983, University Park Press, pp 75-95.

McGlone R, Hollien H: Vocal pitch characteristics of aged women, *J Speech Hear Res* 6:164-170, 1963.

Michel J, Hollien H, Moore P: Speaking fundamental frequency characteristics of 15-, 16-, and 17 year-old girls, *Lang Speech* 9:46-51, 1966.

Miller MA: Speech and voice patterns associated with hearing impairment, *Audecibel* 17:162-167, 1968.

Monsen RB: Durational aspects of vowel production in the speech of deaf children, *J Speech Hear Res* 17:386-398, 1974.

Mysak EE: Pitch and duration characteristics of older males, *J Speech Hear Res* 2:46-59, 1959.

Nickerson RS: Characteristics of the speech of deaf persons, *Volta Rev* 77:342-362, 1975.

Nickerson RS, Steven KN, Boothroyd A et al: Some observations on timing in the speech of deaf and hearing speakers, *BBN Rep No. 2905*, 1974.

Osberger MJ, Levitt H: The effect of timing errors on the intelligibility of deaf children's speech, *J Acoust Soc Am* 66:1316-1324, 1979.

Owens E, Telleen C: Speech perception with hearing aids and cochlear implants, *Arch Otolaryngol* 107:160-163, 1981.

Parkhurst BG, Levitt H: The effect of selected prosodic errors on the intelligibility of deaf speakers, *J Comm Dis* 11:249-256, 1978.

Penn G: Voice and speech patterns in the hard of hearing, *Acta Otolaryngol* 124(Suppl):1-69, 1955.

Plant G: The effects of an acquired profound hearing loss on speech production, *Br J Aud* 18:39-48, 1984.

Ramsden RT: Rehabilitation of the suddenly deafened adult, *Ear Nose Throat J*, 60:49-54, 1981.

Silverman SR, Calvert DR: Conservation and development of speech. In Davis H, Silverman SR, editors: *Hearing and deafness*, New York, 1978, Holt, Rhinehart, & Winston, pp 388-399.

Smith CR: Residual hearing and speech production in deaf children, *J Speech Hear Res* 18:795-811, 1975.

Stark RE, Levitt H: Prosodic feature perception and production in deaf children, *J Acoust Soc Am* 55:63, 1974 (abstract).

Stoicheff ML: Speaking fundamental frequency characteristics of nonsmoking female adults, *J Speech Hear Res* 24:437-441, 1981.

Tong YC, Clark GM, Blamey PJ et al: Psychophysical studies for two multiple channel cochlear implantations, *J Acous Soc Am* 71:153-160, 1982.

Tye N, Zimmermann GN, Kelso JAS: Compensatory articulation in hearing impaired speakers: a cine-fluorographic study, *J Phonetics* 11:101-115, 1983.

Voelker CH: A preliminary strobophotoscopic study of the speech of the deaf, *Am Ann Deaf* 80:243-259, 1935.

Voelker CH: An experimental study of the comparative rate of utterance of deaf and normal speakers, *Am Ann Deaf* 83:274-284, 1938.

Zimmermann G, Collins MJ: The speech of the adventitiously deaf and auditory information: a reply to Goehl and Kaufman (1984), *J Speech Hear Dis* 50:220-221, 1985.

Zimmermann G, Rettaliata P: Articulatory patterns of an adventitiously deaf speaker: implications for the role of auditory information in speech production, *J Speech Hear Res* 24:169-178, 1981.

CHAPTER **6**

Applications and Resources

Most clinicians agree that modifying patient/client behavior in the therapy situation is only an intermediate goal of rehabilitation. Ultimately, we should strive for improved behavior and performance *outside of the clinic* in the various locations and conditions that make up real life. The two most important environments for improvement are the *home* and the *workplace;* therefore, they merit special discussion. It must be acknowledged, however, that for a given deafened individual, improved interaction with medical caregivers (typifying an intimate one-to-one exchange) or communication in a religious setting (exemplifying a group situation) may be of paramount importance; therefore, some comments about these situations will be included in the following sections.

HOME MILIEU

The home environment may be the greatest challenge for the patient. Success here requires modification of the home's physical properties and use of appropriate assistive devices. Moreover, it requires modification of behavior of the patient and of significant others, some of whom may not have attended counseling with the hearing-impaired person.

The physical arrangement of the home should be reviewed. In order to do this properly, the audiologist or counselor may need to visit the home or have access to a detailed floor plan. The description should be detailed in terms of characteristics that affect reverberation time, such as presence of carpeting, draperies, and surface materials. The number of rooms and levels, location of telephone and extensions, arrangement of television and seating, placement of front door and other entrances, and the manner in which the spaces are used are influential in advising the family about application of information presented in therapy.

Sometimes, the hearing-impaired person resists making home modifications. For example:

In our patient caseload, J.M., a 67-year-old man with bilateral complete hearing loss, had also experienced bilateral above-the-knee amputations and at least one cerebrovascular accident. He accepted his family's renovation of his house to include multiple ramps and other modifications for wheelchair accessibility. However, he steadfastly refused the installation of alerting devices, or consistent use of his vibrotactile device or TDD. When questioned about his reasoning, he simply stated that he had been deaf a long time, and "Who would call me, anyway?" He acknowledged that he might want to be able to use the TDD for emergency calls but still considered it acceptable to rely on his wife for all telephone communication and detection of visitors at the front door.

It is not appropriate to force modifications on any individual, yet the objective of much of what we do is to increase independence. To the fullest extent possible, the clinician should help the patient examine the source of resistance to change and to accept that accommodations are desirable.

The patient and family, after the informational counseling (outlined more fully in Chapter 2), should understand in general the types of assistive devices that are available but may still need specific guidance about applying the devices in their environment. In some homes, a flashing light connected to the doorbell or flashing lamps may suffice; in others, a vibrotactile alerting device using FM transmitters from multiple locations may be necessary. While installation of a television decoder may be the sole appropriate recommendation for a late-deafened adult with profound loss, an individual with severe hearing loss should be advised about maximizing auditory input as well as using the visual channel. Such mechanisms as an FM ALD or direct audio input should be considered, in most instances *along with* a caption decoder.

Ideally, a trial in the home with such an arrangement for television should be undertaken, as different persons may experience various levels of success, depending on auditory factors (e.g., speech discrimination in quiet, recognition ability in a reverberant room), nonauditory characteristics (e.g., closure ability, figure-ground discrimination, knowledge of the language being broadcast), and acoustic influences (e.g., reverberation, background noise, clarity of the acoustic signal broadcast). Similarly, other alerting devices or ALDs should undergo a trial in the home (or other intended setting) whenever feasible.

The clinician's suggestions for improvement of the home environment may be "low-tech." Alteration of background noise levels or competing signals (from noisy home equipment such as dishwashers or air conditioner/heating sources) may be suggested. Use of sound-absorptive materials (including draperies and carpeting), rearrangement of furniture, or improved lighting for speechreading may all be low cost/high yield improvements in improving the home's accessibility for communication.

Issues surrounding maximal adjustment in the home situation involve both habit and intimacy. Often, the hearing-impaired adult and family or significant others have experienced communication with each other—with various levels of success or failure—over many years. The subtle habits developed in these interactions are difficult to examine objectively, even in the light of newly gained insights obtained through counseling. For example:

S.E. came to our program alone. He was found to have complete sensorineural hearing loss bilaterally. He described his loss as gradual in onset and of unknown origin. He lived with his son in an apartment in Brooklyn. According to S.E., he had not exchanged "a word with anybody for [the last] 3 years."

Such abject isolation is an extreme example of the loss of contact with a significant other, in this case, a son. Certainly, a lesser degree of hearing loss or lesser extent of isolation may, nonetheless, be acutely painful.

Common complaints, heard by clinicians from patients with all degrees of hearing loss, involve actions that are implicitly irrational:

For example, P.R. (a male with severe hearing loss) complained that his wife routinely called him when she was in the basement pantry and he was on the first floor of their home. "She always asks me things like 'Do you want a can of peas?'" he complained. "Does she expect me to understand her? Peas? Beets? I don't know!" His wife, on the other hand, replied that she knew he could not understand something like that, but she also couldn't be expected to walk up and down each time a question arose. Their anger escalated to a point where they went for days, exchanging only bare verbal necessities.

Modifying behavior for such a couple in the clinic is inadequate; the habit of speaking from another level (or room) is deeply ingrained in people who have lived together a long time. The inconvenience entailed in the demanded face-to-face communication at a short distance is a powerful negative motivator. Similarly, supplying a family group with assistive devices alone is also an incomplete answer. They must identify their irrational communication actions and alter behavior.

As Rocky Stone, the founder of Self-Help for the Hard of Hearing (SHHH) has pointed out (Trace, 1992), hearing loss interferes with the normal communication processes needed to develop or maintain intimacy. Living together is clearly no guarantee of intimate, mutual understanding. As with the couple described previously, anger may result in limited exchanges and deterioration of the relationship. Thus the importance of communication for intimacy in the home environment cannot be underestimated. As the couple or family unit undergoes psychologic and communication counseling, the audiologist may promote improved communication in the home by using appropriate devices and techniques.

One practical suggestion for enhanced communication in the home is the use of direct audio input to either an auditory (powerful hearing aid or FM auditory trainer/ALD), vibrotactile, or implant device. The benefit of such an arrangement goes beyond improved auditory stimulation for the hearing-impaired person. Direct audio input also requires the significant other to use a device, to focus more on the act of communication. In a hard-wire arrangement, the significant other is required to hold or be attached to a microphone at a distance dictated by the connecting cord. Speechreading is thus enhanced by the more direct, closer visual contact.

The family should also be encouraged to use the old standby, the paper pad and pencil. The intent is to write key words or words with poor visibility, not as a substitute for speechreading, but as a means of reducing stress in the home situation, especially during conversations conveying critical family information. If the family and deafened adult are amenable to learning fingerspelling or selected signs, an overall aural/oral environment may be enhanced by the occasional spelling or signing of a difficult word or phrase, again moving toward reduced communication stress in the home.

In a similar manner, when the late-deafened adult is about to enter into an intimate communication situation, such as a meeting with a physician, preparation is the key to success. This is a prime example of a situation in which the hearing-impaired adult must apply what has been learned in assertive behavior and communication strategies. It is necessary when beginning a session with such a professional to set the stage (i.e., inform the other member of the dyad of the degree of loss or reliance on lipreading), indicate the best means for communicating, request the use of an assistive device, and ask for written clarification as needed. This type of intimate session is the ideal circumstance for applying the assertive behaviors listed in Table 2-4 and the repair strategies described in Chapter 4. Without these steps, there is risk of inadequate information transfer concerning health status, improper use of medications, or other misapplications of professional instructions or guidance. When such breakdowns in intimate communications occur, the significant other may be brought in to supplant the deafened adult as the object of this interaction. Such affronts to the independence of the hearing-impaired adult are avoidable in most cooperative situations by proper use of assertive techniques and assistive devices.

An additional possible loss of intimacy can occur because some hearing-impaired persons are unable to control vocal loudness. In addition to losing the privacy needed to discuss personal issues, there is often a misinterpretation by the listener that excessive or widely fluctuating loudness indicates hostile or agressive intentions. Fear of making such errors in vocal intensity often is the reason that a hearing-impaired adult is reticent to engage in intimate discussions with professionals. Use of the practice techniques discussed in Chapter 5 may lessen embarrassment associated with such voice abnormalities.

It must also be acknowledged that, sometimes, the hearing-impaired adult will encounter uncooperative, poor communicators who may be reluctant or unable to change their patterns of interaction to cope with a hearing-impaired individual. If the deafened adult is insistent in these circumstances, the other person may become recalcitrant or, possibly, adversarial. If that occurs, the sought-after intimacy is clearly defeated. Ideally, both parties should seek a comfortable communication compromise.

WORK ENVIRONMENT

Accommodations for the hearing impaired in the workplace are (as discussed in Chapter 1) mandated by law. The Americans with Disabilities Act (ADA) indicates that an employer is obligated to make *reasonable accommodation* for an individual with a disability. The law does not require that the employer make such adjustments or purchase such devices as to create an undue (financial) hardship. It is also incumbent on the employer to provide accommodation to prevent the disabled employee from posing a direct threat to his/her own safety or that of other persons at the job site (DeWine, 1992).

Education of the public, in general, and of potential employers of the hearing impaired is a worthy long-term goal of speech and hearing professionals. At this time, most employers have only limited (or no) understanding of the devices that are available to improve access to their hearing-impaired employees. Thus an employer is likely to need professional consultation in order to make proper accommodations. In addition, an employee who is having job-related problems may request that a member(s) of the rehabilitation team advise the employer about reasonable adjustments in the workplace to enhance employee performance and ensure improved safety.

In manufacturing settings, noise interferes with all forms of routine communication. Warnings regarding potentially dangerous situations are frequently announced by loudspeaker or siren. A supervisor may shout an instruction to an employee from a distance. In the noisy job situation, reception (for a person with some residual hearing) is clearly impaired. For the adult with a complete hearing loss, the presence of noise does not further reduce their (already nil auditory) reception of speech, although it must be acknowledged that noise may reach the level of physical discomfort for them as well as for persons with normal hearing or lesser levels of hearing impairment. This possibility of discomfort is especially great for persons with sensorineural loss accompanied by recruitment.

The challenge in this environment is to present a recognizable alerting signal that will move the worker's visual attention from his/her job task to potential source(s) of danger or to another person trying to make visual contact to initiate communication. One especially useful assistive device in a noisy industrial setting is a vibrotactile pager. The wearer can be alerted to divert attention to scan the environment visually, or can be given a specific message if the pager has text capability. A less expensive approach may be to wire a flashing signal or color-coded light array to the deafened adult's work station to convey prearranged messages.

The hearing-impaired employee in such a work setting may have to assert his/her desire to have job-related conferences with the supervisor in a private location. There is a temptation for the supervisor to raise the loudness of his/her voice to compensate for the background noise level. Work conferences should take place under conditions that permit the employee to request use of an ALD, repetition of spoken messages, or written confirmation of information. Implementation of communication rights suggested by Vaughn (1986) (see Chapter 2, Appendix G) is clearly appropriate in such interviews.

For the office worker, the devices needed for reasonable accommodation may be more varied. In addition to certain alerting aids, as described previously, it may be necessary to obtain devices for facilitating communication over the telephone, including TDDs and telefax machines. In the severely and profoundly impaired group, telephone amplifiers coupled to the tele-coil of a contemporary personal hearing aid are seldom sufficient for accurate information transfer. As Cranmer-Briskey (1992) points out, the new legislation is expected to increase demand for tele-coils of improved quality, possibly increasing their utility at least for the severely impaired adult.

Other accommodations in the office may include use of assistive listening devices (FM, infrared, induction loop, or hard-wire) and videotext displays or transcription, supplemented by prepared printed text of lectures or presentations. In addition, certified interpreters or notetakers should be used as appropriate. When audio-taped training materials are used, written text should be supplied for hearing-impaired employees. Videotapes should be prepared with closed or open captions; this suggestion is only feasible for large companies, otherwise the expense would undoubtedly be considered an undue hardship.

Similar challenges and options are available for a congregant who seeks to improve participation in religious services. It is feasible to request that clergy provide a text of a sermon or other speech in advance of the actual presentation; many religious leaders will be pleased to do so. Such accommodations as were discussed for the workplace (ranging in cost from under a hundred dollars to several thousands) may not present an insurmountable obstacle for purchase by the congregation. This is especially reasonable when it is recognized that the late-deafened adult may not be the sole hearing-impaired person in the group. Although several other congregants may be hearing impaired to a lesser degree, the profoundly impaired adult may be able to make use of a system that can be tuned to the needs of several individual users. Consultation with an audiologist or engineer specializing in group systems is warranted before purchase by the organization.

Some public venues, such as theaters, have already purchased communication aids and make them available for rental by their clientele. However, devices used in such environments may not meet the need of some adults with a profound hearing loss. It may be worthwhile to experiment to find out if a device is useful in a particular theater, but it is also necessary to recognize an ALD may simply not overcome the barrier imposed by a difficult listening and lipreading situation.

Years of experience may be needed before employers or other organizations become well-versed in the methods of complying with the requirements and intents of the ADA. Many of the resources listed in this chapter are not well-known within the professional community, let alone the broader populace.

LISTING OF RESOURCES

The following section is divided into two listings (not in order of importance): (1) some of the numerous resources that are available for late-deafened adults and their families and (2) sources for test and therapy materials for the professional. It is a vital aspect of counseling to increase awareness of such services and groups and the means to obtain assistive devices.

In the following listing, telephone lines may be specified as available for voice communication (V) or for receipt of TDD calls (TDD). That information is listed immediately after the telephone number.

RESOURCES FOR THE PROFOUNDLY HEARING-IMPAIRED ADULT AND FAMILY
Self-Help Groups

Association for Late-Deafened Adults (ALDA)
P.O. Box 641763
Chicago, IL 60664-1763
(312)604-4192 (TDD)
(312)604-5209 (Telefax)

Cochlear Implant Club International
P.O. Box 464
Buffalo, NY 14223-0464
(716)838-4662 (V/TDD)

Self-Help for the Hard of Hearing (SHHH)
7800 Wisconsin Avenue
Bethesda, MD 20814
(301)657-2248 (V)
(301)657-2249 (TDD)

Suzanne Pathy Speak-Up Institute
525 Park Avenue
New York, NY 10021
(No business phone)

Telecommunications for the Deaf
814 Thayer Avenue
Silver Spring, MD 20910
(301)589-3006 (TDD)
(301)589-3786 (V)

Veterans Organization for the Hearing Impaired (VOHI) (founding chapter)
Audiology and Speech Pathology Service/126
VA Medical Center
9600 North Point Road
Fort Howard, MD 21052-3018
(301)687-8852/3 (V)

State or Federal Agencies

Converse/TDD Mediator
(800)842-9910

Connecticut Commission for the Deaf and Hearing-Impaired (name varies in
    different states; may provide referral for specialized services [such as psychol-
    ogists experienced in working with the hearing impaired, interpreter ser-
    vices]; in some states may be a source of assistive devices)

Department of Veterans Affairs (provides services to eligible veterans through
    their local medical center or outpatient clinic)
Audiology and Speech Pathology Service/126CO
VA Medical Center
50 Irving Street, N.W.
Washington, D.C. 20422
(202)745-8578 (V)

Department of Vocational or Rehabilitation Services (name varies from state to
    state; may provide [re]training for adults of employable age)

Food and Drug Administration (FDA) (regulates devices for the hearing im-
    paired, such as cochlear implants and hearing aids)
5600 Fisher's Lane
Rockville, MD 20852
(301)443-1544

National Captioning Institute (NCI) (provides information on television closed
captioning and decoders)
5203 Leesburg Pike
Falls Church, VA 22041
(703)998-2416

National Institutes of Deafness and Communicative Disorders (NIDCD) (oper-
ates a clearinghouse for information about hearing, balance, smell, taste,
voice, speech, and language)
National Institutes of Health and Human Services
Building 31, Room 3C-35
9000 Rockville Pike
Bethesda, MD 20892
(301) 496-7243 (V)
(301) 402-0018 (TDD)

Private Organizations

Alexander Graham Bell Association for the Deaf (offers a variety of educational
materials, some of which are appropriate for adults [e.g., Castle, DL "Signaling and assistive devices for hearing-impaired people"])
3417 Volta Place, N.W.
Washington, D.C. 20007
(202) 337-5220

AMVETS (national organization of veterans; local chapters may support various projects at a VA medical center, including providing assistance to
nonservice-connected veterans by some chapters)

American Academy of Otolaryngology (AAOO) (provides information about
hearing loss and treatment)
1101 Vermont Avenue, N.W.
Washington, D.C. 20005
(202)289-4607

American Speech-Language-Hearing Association (ASHLA) (provides information about hearing loss and referral sources for ASHLA-certified programs)
10801 Rockville Pike
Rockville, MD 20852
(800)638-6868

AT&T Operator for the Deaf (assistance in placing calls to other TDDs)
(800)855-1155

Boy's Town National Institute for Communication Disorders in Children
555 North 30th Street
Omaha, NE 68131
(402)449-6540 (V)
(402)449-6543 (TDD)

Central Institute for the Deaf (CID)
Hearing, Language, and Speech Clinic
818 South Euclid
St. Louis, MO 63112
(314)652-3200 (V)
(314)533-9857 (TDD)

Clarke School for the Deaf
Round Hill Road
Northampton, MA 01060-2199
(413)584-3450 (V/TDD)

Consumers Organization for the Hearing Impaired
P.O. Box 8188
Silver Spring, MD 20907

Deafness Research Foundation (provides grant support for research projects re-
    lated to the ear)
9 East 38th Street
New York, NY 10016
(212)684-6556

National Information Center on Deafness
Gallaudet University
800 Florida Avenue, N.E.
Washington, D.C. 20001-3625
(202)651-5051

HEAR Now (provides financial assistance to a limited number of applicants for
    cochlear implant support)
4001 South Magnolia Way, Suite 100
Denver, CO 80237
(303)758-4919
(800)648-HEAR (V/TDD)

Job Accommodation Network (JAN) (provides information about means to solve communication problems in a work environment; affiliated with Gallaudet Assistive Devices Center)
P.O. 468
Morgantown, WV 26505
(800)526-7234
[(800)526-4698, West Virginia only]

Lions' Club (National service organization with local chapters; as part of community service, Lions chapters may support various capital investments in equipment for an aural rehabilitation program; individuals may be sponsored for special projects, such as the purchase of an assistive device by a local chapter)

National Technical Institute for the Deaf at Rochester Institute of Technology (produces research and publications about deafness and training strategies)
One Lomb Memorial Drive
P.O. Box 9887
Rochester, NY 14623
(716)475-6400

Organization for the Use of the Telephone (OUT)
P.O. Box 175
Owings Mills, MD 21117

Sertoma (national service organization with local chapters; as part of community service, Sertoma chapters may support various capital investments in equipment for an aural rehabilitation program)
1912 East Meyer Boulevard
P.O. Box 17003
Kansas City, MO 64119-1174
(816)333-8300

Tele-Consumer Hotline (assists consumers in telephone shopping activities)
1536 16th Street, N.W.
Washington, D.C. 20036
(800)332-1124

Distributors of Assistive Devices*

AT&T National Special Needs Center
2001 Route 46 East
Parsippany, NJ 07054-1315
(800)233-1222

---

*The manufacturers and distributors of ALDs are numerous and constantly changing. Therefore our list may not be exhaustive. It is advisable to consult the annual directories provided by technical publications, such as *Hearing Instruments* and *Hearing Journal*.

Audex (manufacturer and distributor of ALDs)
713 North Fourth Street
Longview, TX 75601
(800)237-0716

Audio Enhancement (national distributor of Comtek wireless auditory assistance kits)
8 Winfield Point Lane
St. Louis, MO 63141
(314)567-6141

Audiological Engineering (manufacturer of Tactaid 2 and Tactaid 7)
9 Preston
Sommerville, MA 02143
(617)623-5562 (V)
(800)283-4601 (V)
(800)955-7204 (TDD)

Audiotone
P.O. Box 2905
Phoenix, AZ 85062
(602)254-5886

Canine Companions for Independence (one of several such training facilities throughout the country)
P.O. Box 446
Santa Rosa, CA 95402
(707)579-1985

Cochlear Corporation (U.S. distributor of the Nucleus multichannel cochlear implant; provider of repairs and supplies for House single-channel cochlear implant)
61 Inverness Drive East
Suite 100
Englewood, CO 80112
(303)790-9010
(800)523-5798

Deaf Products (offers a variety of assistive and alterting devices)
P.O. Box 2256
Costa Mesa, CA 92628-2256
(714)549-5123 (V/TDD)

Dogs for the Deaf (one of several such training facilities throughout the country)
10175 Wheeler Road
Central Point, OR 97502
(503)826-9220 (V/TDD)

Earmark
1125 Dixwell Avenue
Hamden, CT 06514
(203)777-2130

Hal-Hen Company
P.O. Box 6077
Long Island City, NY 11106-9990
(718)392-6020

HARC Mercantile Ltd.
3130 Portage
P.O. Box 3055
Kalamazoo, MI 49003-3055
(616)381-0177 (V)
(800)445-9968 (V)
(616)381-2219 (TDD)

Harris Communications
Dept. VOI A/S 91
3255 Hennepin Avenue, Suite 55
Minneapolis, MN 55408
(800)825-6758 (V)
(800)825-9187 (TDD)

Hearing Ear Dog Program (provides information and support to obtain hearing ear dogs from local specialized trainers)
P.O. Box 213
West Boylston, MA 01583
(508)835-3304 (V/TDD)

House Ear Institute (offers publications about ear disorders and medical treatment, such as "Understanding Acoustic Tumors," "Understanding Tinnitus")
2100 West Third Street
Los Angeles, CA 90057
(213)483-4431

Krown Research, Inc.
6300 Arizona Circle
Los Angeles, CA 90045
(213)641-4306 (V)
(800)344-3277 (TDD)

Mini-Med Technologies (manufacturer of a multichannel cochlear implant associated with the research conducted at the University of California at San Francisco: at the time of this writing, this device is investigational)
12744 San Fernando Road
Sylmar, CA 91342
(818)362-5958 (V)
(800)933-3322 (V)

National Catalog House of the Deaf (supplier of many assistive and alerting devices)
4300 North Kilpatrick Avenue
Chicago, IL 60641
(312)283-2907 (V)

National Hearing Aid Distributors, Inc.
a/k/a The Source
145 Tremont Street
Boston, MA 02111
(617)426-9845 (V)
(617)426-7023 (TDD)
(800)627-9930 (V)

Oticon Corporation
29 Schoolhouse Road, P.O. 6724
Somerset, NJ 08875-6724
(908)560-1220 (V)
(800)526-3921

Phonic Ear
250 Camino Alto
Mill Valley, CA 94941
(800)227-0735

Precision Controls, Inc.
5 Thomas South
Hawthorne, NJ 07506
(201)423-3475

Radio Shack, Inc. (has a variety of hardware that can be used in combination with television, radio, telephone, or for construction of loop systems)
300 One Tandy Center
Fort Worth, TX 76102
(817)390-3011 (V)

Red Acre Farm (one of several such training facilities throughout the country)
Hearing Dog Center
109 Red Acre Road
Stow, MA
(508)897-8343

Sears, Roebuck and Company (sells closed caption decoder adapters and combination units with television)
Sears Tower
Chicago, IL

Siemens Hearing Instruments, Inc.
10 Corporate Place South
Piscataway, NJ 08854
(800)345-0183

Silent Call Corporation
P.O. Box 16348
Clarkston, MI 48106-6348
(313)391-1710

Smith and Nephew Richards, Inc. (manufacturers of the device formerly known as the Utah or Symbion cochlear implant)
ATT: Cochlear Implant Department
2925 Appling Road
Bartlett, TN 38133
(800)821-5700

Sonic Alert (offers a variety of signaling devices)
1750 West Hamlin Road
Rochester Hill, MI 48309
(313)656-3110

Sonovation Inc. (produces an FM ALD with a behind-the-ear receiver/hearing aid)
4116 Cedar Avenue
Minneapolis, MN 55407
(612)721-2129

Sound Resources, Inc.
210 Odgen
Hinsdale, IL 60521
(312)323-6133

Speech and Hearing Technologies (speechreading counseling videotapes)
480 Queensgate Road
Springboro, OH 45066

Telex Communications, Inc.
9600 Aldrich Avenue, South
Minneapolis, MN 55420
(800)328-8212

Wheelock Signals, Inc.
273 Branport Avenue
Long Branch, NJ 07740
(201)222-6880

Williams Sound Corp.
5929 Baker Road
Minnetonka, MN 55345-5997
(800)328-6190

Publications

ALDA News (official newsletter of the Association for Late-Deafened Adults, Chicago Style; see earlier entry)

CICI (publication of the Cochlear Implant Club International; see earlier entry)

SHHH Magazine (official publication of Self-Help for the Hard of Hearing; see earlier entry)

Hearing Health—The Voice on Hearing Health
P.O. Box 2663
Corpus Christi, TX 78403-2663
(512)884-8388 (V/TDD)

SOURCES FOR THE PROFESSIONAL

Academy of Dispensing Audiologists (offers videotape and companion book, *Assistive Devices: Doorways to Independence)*
3008 Millwood Avenue
Columbia, SC 29205
(803)252-5646

Auditec of St. Louis (offers copies of Minimal Auditory Capabilities Battery, connected discourse, multi-talker noise, cafeteria noise, tele-coil evaluation procedure, sound effects recognition test, CID sentences)
330 Selma Avenue
St. Louis, MO 63119
(314)962-5890

Cochlear Corporation (offers copies of BKB Sentences, Speech Pattern Contrast Test; see earlier entry)

Foreworks (produces Test of Auditory Comprehension)
P.O. Box 9747
North Hollywood, CA 91609

National Acoustics Laboratory (NAL) (produces many rehabilitative materials, including COMMTRAM, COMMTRAC, and SYNTREX)
ATT: The Marketing Officer
126 Greyville Street
Chatswood, New South Wales 2067
Australia

National Institutes of Deafness and Communicative Disorders (NIDCD, see earlier entry for address; provides research funding regarding biomedical and behavioral problems associated with communication impairments or disorders; grants offered for individual, institutional, career development; center grants and contracts to public and private research facilities; research efforts in the development of therapeutic interventions and devices are supported)

New York League for the Hard of Hearing (produces educational materials, such as videotapes for lipreading self-instruction—"I See What You're Saying" and "Assistive Devices for Hearing-Impaired Persons")
71 West 23 Street
New York, New York 10010
(212)741-3144 (Voice)
(212)741-1932 (TDD)

Sign Enhancers, Inc. (produces videotapes on ASL and deaf awareness)
1913 Rockland Drive, N.W.
Salem, Or 97304
(503)370-9721 (TDD)

The University of Iowa Hospital (offers copies of Sentence Without Context Test, Medial Consonant Nonsense Syllables Test, both auditory and video-tape versions)
Audiology Section
Department of Otolaryngology
Iowa City, IA 52242
(319)356-2471

REFERENCES

Cranmer-Briskey KS: The ADA spells urgency for telecoil use, *Hear Instru* 43(8):8-12, 1992.
DeWine L: Americans with Disabilities Act: a declaration of opportunities, *Audecibel* July/August/September, pp 7-10, 1992.
Trace R: Hearing loss and sexuality, *Advance Speech-Lang Pathol Audiol* 7, June 1, 1992.
Vaughn GR: Bill of rights for listeners and talkers, *Hear Instru* 37:8, 1986.

Index